a **parent's** guide to

intuitive
eating

how to raise kids
who love to eat healthy

Dr. Yami Cazorla-Lancaster DO, MPH, MS, FAAP

⊖ ULYSSES PRESS

Published in the United States by:
ULYSSES PRESS
P.O. Box 3440
Berkeley, CA 94703
www.ulyssespress.com

ISBN: 978-1-61243-933-4
Library of Congress Control Number: 2019905489

Printed in the United States by Kingery Printing Company
10 9 8 7 6 5 4 3 2 1

Acquisitions editor: Casie Vogel
Managing editor: Claire Chun
Editor: Renee Rutledge
Proofreader: Ruby Privateer
Index: S4Carlisle Publishing Services
Front cover design: Justin Shirley
Cover photo: © travelarium.photos
Interior design: what!design @ whatweb.com
Production: Jake Flaherty

NOTE TO READERS: This book has been written and published strictly for informational and educational purposes only. It is not intended to serve as medical advice or to be any form of medical treatment. You should always consult your physician before altering or changing any aspect of your medical treatment and/or undertaking a diet regimen, including the guidelines as described in this book. Do not stop or change any prescription medications without the guidance and advice of your physician. Any use of the information in this book is made on the reader's good judgment after consulting with his or her physician and is the reader's sole responsibility. This book is not intended to diagnose or treat any medical condition and is not a substitute for a physician.

This book is independently authored and published and no sponsorship or endorsement of this book by, and no affiliation with, any trademarked brands or other products mentioned within is claimed or suggested. All trademarks that appear in ingredient lists and elsewhere in this book belong to their respective owners and are used here for informational purposes only. The author and publisher encourage readers to patronize the quality brands mentioned and pictured in this book.

"Dr. Yami Cazorla-Lancaster has written a book for parents that promotes love, compassion, and acceptance as the foundation for feeding their children. She believes wholeheartedly in the principles of Intuitive Eating and Health at Every Size and is committed to showing you the way to bring up your children to have a healthy relationship with food and their bodies. She helps parents heal their own relationships with food, so that they are able to teach their children to trust their inner wisdom about eating. Although Dr. Yami has a preference for plant-based foods, her goal is to encourage the inclusion of these foods for their health benefits, without prescribing this way of eating as an all-or-nothing approach. If you're confused by all the conflicting messages about feeding your child, this book will lead you along the path of peace, joy, and nourishment for your child and your family."

> —Elyse Resch, MS, RDN, CEDRD-S, FAND
> Author of *The Intuitive Eating Workbook for Teens*
> Coauthor of *Intuitive Eating* and *The Intuitive Eating Workbook*

"Dr. Yami's book provides parents with a complete guide for raising healthy children from pregnancy to late childhood. She underscores the importance of providing children with well-rounded meals filled with fruits, vegetables, beans, and whole grains, along with covering topics such as picky eating, body image, and important lifestyle habits. You won't want to miss this comprehensive resource!"

> —Neal Barnard, MD, FACC
> President, Physicians Committee for Responsible Medicine

"Children need guidance in making healthy food choices—and so do their parents! *A Parent's Guide to Intuitive Eating* integrates Yami's pediatric expertise with relevant personal experiences. No matter your age, or the age of your child, this book will guide you toward eating a healthy, satisfying diet—that will be sustainable through life."

> —Dreena Burton
> Author of *Plant-Powered Families*
> www.dreenaburton.com

"Dr. Yami nailed it and at the same time set us free. This book reorients us to our lost superpower—eating! ... and the healthiest way to do so. Raising plant-based kiddos gives the whole family a leg up on health and well-being. A parental must read."

> —Jane Esselstyn, RN
> Coauthor of *The Prevent and Reverse Heart Disease Cookbook: Over 125 Delicious, Life-Changing, Plant-Based Recipes*

"Dr. Yami is a truly compassionate and incredible pediatrician. Her guide on intuitive eating for children is a fresh and honest approach to combatting the serious childhood obesity epidemic plaguing our world. As a mother of three myself and a physician I would highly recommend this book to anyone who wants their children to grow up healthy and free of chronic disease. Thank you, Dr. Yami!"

> —Laurie Marbas, MD, MBA
> Cofounder, HealthyHumanRevolution.com

"An essential guide full of important information for raising children healthfully. Dr. Yami shows us that when we start to focus on living for health and joy rather than for body weight, something magical happens. We are freed from our stressful relationship with food and begin to make choices that align with our family values and health goals."

> —Beth Motley, MD
> Family Medicine/Lifestyle Medicine

"In a world where there is so much confusion about nutrition, Dr. Yami provides a delightful guide full of information for those of us who want to enjoy eating healthy food and raising healthy children."

> —Angie Sadeghi, MD, Diplomate,
> American Board of Gastroenterology and
> American Board of Internal Medicine

"Dr. Yami lays out a persuasive case for intuitive eating to set babies and children up for a lifetime of healthy eating. As a new parent and physician, I find the book an invaluable resource already."

> —Heather Shenkman, MD
> Author of *The Vegan Heart Doctor's Guide to Reversing Heart Disease, Losing Weight, and Reclaiming Your Life*

To Kian and Desta, my precious sons and greatest teachers in life. May you find joy in life, take pleasure in food, and accept your beautiful bodies just as they are.

And to my mother, Griselda, my biggest fan and supporter—I love you!

Contents

Introduction

"Trust yourself. You know more than you think you do."

—Benjamin Spock, pediatrician and best-selling author of *The Common Sense Book of Baby and Child Care*

Feeding our children can bring immense joy and incredible stress. We worry that our kids aren't eating enough or that they are eating too much. We become anxious over their growth, wondering if they are too small or too big. We even feel guilty that our kids aren't "good" vegetable eaters or that they prefer carbs to greens. Well-meaning friends and family members may comment on our children's eating habits or body size, sending us into a spiral of doubt and shame. On top of all this, we live in a fast-paced culture that values thinness, and we, as parents, may struggle with our own body image and history of dieting. It's no wonder that mealtime becomes a battle zone for many families, leading to frustration, confusion, and tears for kids and moms alike.

I've experienced every single one of these feelings and been in all of these situations. I might be a pediatrician, but at home, I'm a mom, and I've had to figure it out, sometimes the hard way. I'm grateful that motherhood has taught me some valuable lessons, though it has felt difficult at times. At this point in my career and motherhood, I know one thing for sure—it doesn't have to be so complicated! More great news: You don't have to be perfect! I'll be the first to tell you that I am far from perfect. Parenting has taught me to learn from my mistakes. I've learned that many of the food battles with our children stem from fear. It is trust, patience, and respect that lead to the creation of confident eaters.

Intuitive eating is a philosophy that respects each person as an expert of their hunger and fullness signals. Instead of focusing on food rules, quantities, calories, and strict schedules, it is centered around supporting and guiding your child to navigate internal cues that indicate when, what, and how much to eat. Unfortunately, we aren't great at practicing intuitive eating in the United States because we don't trust ourselves. Much of this mistrust is driven by the desire to fit an ideal body size or to live up to an absolute healthy ideal. We rely on meal plans, fad diets, calorie and macronutrient counting, and other external indicators of when to eat.

Believe me, I've tried all of these approaches before, and I feel fortunate that I found intuitive eating and the Health at Every Size (HAES®)[1] philosophy. Health at Every Size principles emphasize a holistic approach to health, body size acceptance, social justice, and making physical movement and eating choices that are pleasurable and in tune with internal cues. More about this later, but first let me tell you a little bit about how I got here.

My Story

My name is Yamileth Cazorla-Lancaster, also known as "Dr. Yami" to my patients. I am a board-certified pediatrician, mother, health coach, and professional speaker. I'm passionate about the power that our diet and lifestyle habits have on our health, joy, and longevity. I have seen firsthand how these choices can prevent and reverse disease both in my pediatric patients and my coaching clients. I live and breathe nutrition and lifestyle

---

1   Health At Every Size and HAES are registered trademarks of the Association for Size Diversity and Health and used with permission.

medicine because I know how important it is for me, my family, my patients, and my clients.

But I wasn't always this way. I didn't grow up with the healthiest diet. As a child, I was labeled as a "good eater" by my family and was a proud member of the "clean plate club." I loved sugary cereal with whole milk, savored fried foods, and was not picky in the least. When I was in elementary school, I was a latchkey kid. Home alone in the afternoons, I ate for entertainment. I began to suffer from constant tummy aches and constipation. I would often go an entire week between bowel movements. When I did have a bowel movement, it was hard and painful. However, I thought this was normal because everybody in my family suffered from constipation. I never really associated my digestive problems with my diet, and nobody else did either.

As I grew older, my family worried that I was overeating. I went on my first, 1,200-calorie, doctor-prescribed diet at age nine. And it worked—I lost weight. I'll never forget going to the doctor's office for a follow-up and being told that by the next appointment I would be so skinny that he wouldn't be able to see me behind his exam chart. I felt so proud. The validation that I received from losing weight triggered several decades of yo-yo dieting. In junior high, I was bullied by a group of girls who recommended that I go on the SlimFast plan as they giggled. Of course, no diet ever led to the ideal weight and appearance I desired. I spent a lot of days feeling frustrated and depressed about my weight and my body.

My first son was born during my fourth year in medical school. Having a child prompted my interest in nutrition. I was adamant about my son being exposed to a healthy diet and lifestyle. I wanted him to have the best chance possible for a healthy life. But I also felt a lot of anxiety because I didn't want him to grow up "fat" like I did and suffer from bullying or chronic dieting. I was terrified that he would become an overeater like me, and I watched him like a hawk.

My pediatric residency was both an exciting and stressful time in my life. To cope with 80-hour work weeks and chronic sleep deprivation, I developed a vicious binge-eating habit and used food frequently to soothe myself. I was frustrated by the control that food seemed to have in my life, but I couldn't seem to stop.

It wasn't until a few years later that I hit rock bottom. It really should have been the happiest time of my life—I was married to my best friend, I had achieved my lifelong dream of becoming a community pediatrician, and I had a beautiful house and family. My older son was a healthy six-year-old, and we had just adopted our beautiful and joyful second son, who was eighteen months old. But, in spite of all of this, I was miserable. I was anxious, depressed, and unhappy with myself, and my binge eating was out of control. I would vacillate between trying to control every detail of my diet to eating everything in sight. I felt so ashamed by my actions and, even worse, I was irritable with my children and husband. I was also my worst critic.

One day my oldest son, who was around six at the time, started sucking in his stomach and checking his reflection in the mirror frequently. He rapidly developed a self-consciousness about his body that was alarming. It was then that I realized the effect of my behavior. This realization was a huge turning point. I knew that if I didn't address my relationship with my body and food that it could potentially hurt my children and lead to the very issues that I was trying to prevent.

I started working with a life coach who specialized in coaching women with eating disorders, and I learned about intuitive eating and Health at Every Size. I decided that I would stop dieting and weighing myself and, even though it was frightening, it was also incredibly liberating. I found joy in running. My body reached a comfortable equilibrium where I actually started to feel pride in my body without any need to restrict my food or to diet. Food became fun and pleasurable instead of the painful tug-of-war that it had been for so many years.

I also began my journey in plant-based nutrition. Trying a plant-based diet for thirty days as an experiment changed my life. My chronic constipation was cured in just a few days. I felt more energetic, my brain felt calmer, and I had fewer urges to overeat. It would take me another month of research and investigation before I felt reassured that not only was this a safe option for my children, but it was actually health-promoting.

Change is not linear. I wish I could say that as soon as I had this initial breakthrough, I never struggled with food again. It would take several more years of gaining skills, knowledge, and practice to find a comfortable balance and relationship with food, and I admit that I am still learning, growing, and evolving in this area. I have had to develop patience with myself and my children, trusting that even though I am not perfect, everything will be okay.

I have been a practicing pediatrician for over a decade now. The personal experience of growing up as a chubby child and subsequently developing a painful relationship with food and my body has also influenced the way I counsel families. I discuss nutrition and feeding in my office every single day. I find that many parents are anxious and confused. They are frustrated by the way their child eats and worry that they don't eat enough vegetables. These worries often lead to food battles at the dinner table. My discussions with families have taught me so much.

I wrote this book because I wanted to share what I have learned through my education, training, and experience in the hopes that it will help anxious and stressed parents who are trying to do the best they can. I hope that after you read this book you will feel more relaxed, confident, and empowered to feed your child.

This book is organized into four main parts. Part I, How to Eat, is all about the intuitive eating philosophy and how it can be applied to children. We will explore how your own history with food and your body image might influence how you approach feeding your children. I will also explain how to interpret growth charts and discuss the wide range of normal when it comes to body size in children.

In Part II, What to Eat, I delve into the health benefits of whole plant foods. I also discuss how tastes develop and why this is important to remember as your little one acquires taste preferences. In this section, I will provide evidence-based information that will help guide your food choices. But I will also show you how it doesn't have to be all-or-nothing.

In Part III, Setting the Table for Healthy Eating Habits, I discuss lifestyle habits that support healthy eating, such as sleep, exercise, and stress reduction.

In Part IV, Feeding Your Child Through the Years, I go on to discuss some of the differences in feeding children from pregnancy through their high school years. Healthy eating habits begin before your little one is born! Each stage comes with different challenges. I will help you feel prepared for the joys and challenges of each stage of development. I will also discuss special circumstances around food and eating that families commonly encounter, such as social events, eating out, and familial differences.

In the appendix, I review medical conditions, such as illness, overweight, failure to thrive, constipation, ADHD, and other conditions that may change appetite. I also outline signs and symptoms of common eating disorders. Finally, I will present different reasons why you may want to seek professional help.

After you finish this book, you can get started right away and start to ease the tension that may exist at your kitchen table. This is your journey and I feel so grateful and honored to help guide you and walk alongside you on this path to health and joy.

part I

How to Eat

For the most part, healthy young children eat when they're hungry and stop when they're full. Teaching your kids to be in tune with their own hunger and fullness cues will allow them to have a comfortable relationship with food and avoid overeating as they grow older.

—Joy Bauer, nutrition and health expert for *The Today Show*

Chapter 1

Why We
Should Care

Nutrition is a vital component of a healthy and joyful life. It can contribute to health or disease, positively or negatively impacting us in many ways, including well-being and mental health, digestive system function, and athletic performance.

A diet high in processed foods, refined sugars, and other additives can lead to the onset of chronic disease. Physicians are starting to diagnose children with chronic illnesses that are typical for adults, such as metabolic syndrome, type 2 diabetes, and fatty liver disease. Metabolic syndrome is marked by abnormalities in insulin, glucose, or cholesterol, known risk factors for progression to diabetes, heart disease, and fatty liver. According to a literature review by Dr. D. Molnar in 2004, type 2 diabetes accounts for between 8 to 46 percent of all new diabetes diagnoses in children in the United States. It is highly prevalent in some ethnic groups, affecting up to 5 percent of adolescents in Native American tribes. Nonalcoholic fatty liver disease is the most common cause of chronic liver disease in children in the United States. A life burdened with disease threatens to steal health and joy away from our children. But it doesn't have to be this way. We can take a different approach that teaches our children the habits and skills that lead to a health-promoting diet and lifestyle.

Before we set out on starting or changing a behavior or habit, it is helpful to understand *why* we choose to do it. I know you are reading this because you want to raise a healthy child, but what does that really mean? When I make food choices for myself and my children, and when I counsel my patients and families, I have three main goals.

1. Promote Health and Well-Being

The dictionary defines well-being as "the state of being comfortable, healthy, or happy." I want to feel good and I want my family to feel good. I want my children to have plenty of energy, proper digestion, and pain-free bodies. I want to decrease their susceptibility to colds and frequent infections. I want them to enjoy sports and physical activity. I want them to sleep well and regulate their emotions. I want them to feel happy and safe. Essentially this is how I describe "health." Feeling good physically and mentally is something that we can tune into and change rather quickly with our diet and lifestyle choices. Many people start to feel increased energy and improved digestion just days or weeks after making a diet and lifestyle change. Many children live with a state of chronic abdominal pain, constant allergies, depressed mood, and frequent colds. They've lived that way for so long that they may not even remember what it feels like to feel good. My first goal is to promote health and well-being so that children genuinely feel good and can focus on enjoying their childhood.

2. Decrease Risk of Chronic Disease and Support Longevity

My second goal, and one of my great passions, is to decrease the risk of chronic disease and support longevity. This one is harder to stay excited about because it is a very long-term project. Even with poor diet and lifestyle choices, many humans may not be diagnosed with chronic disease until their thirties (even though they may have had symptoms of illness for many years before that). Besides, making choices that may enable us to live to a hundred years and beyond is not usually motivating to children. However, for adults who have experienced serious illness or lost a loved one to a chronic disease, such as heart disease, diabetes, or cancer, prevention can become a strong motivator. The good news is that the majority of chronic disease can be prevented by the choices that we make today and every day. In fact, 80 to 90 percent of chronic diseases can be prevented with diet and lifestyle choices. The key is to develop and foster routines and habits so that they become a way of life and not a burden or a source of suffering.

3. Foster Confidence

My third goal is to help children develop a healthy relationship with food and foster confidence in their bodies. Having suffered from disordered eating and poor body image for many years, I know how painful it can be and how much it can detract from a joyful life. Disordered eating is defined as abnormal eating behaviors that by themselves do not constitute an eating disorder, but include practices such as restricting food or food groups, induced vomiting, and binge eating. Those that have disordered eating are at increased risk for developing an eating disorder. The risk of death for those suffering from eating disorders is significantly elevated. Even if the eating disorder does not result in death, it can cause serious medical complications such as low heart rate, heart palpitations, low blood pressure, muscle wasting, dental erosions, and chronic digestive irregularities. Also, dieting, unhealthy weight-control practices, and binge eating can cause harm—even if they do not meet criteria for eating disorders. Children who start these behaviors as adolescents are likely to continue them into adulthood. If we ourselves become confident and relaxed around food, our food choices, and our bodies, we will give our kids a better chance of learning and adopting these skills as well.

Chapter 2

Intuitive Eating:
Your Child's Superpower

What is intuitive eating, and how can we leverage it? The general concept of intuitive eating has been around since the '70s, but the term was coined in 1995 by authors Evelyn Tribole and Elyse Resch in their groundbreaking book, *Intuitive Eating: A Revolutionary Program That Works*. Tribole and Resch describe an intuitive eater as someone who "honors their hunger, respects their fullness, and enjoys the pleasure of eating." For intuitive eaters, the trigger to eat is physical hunger, the physiological urge to eat prompted by a physical cue such as a growling stomach or a feeling of emptiness in the stomach. It does not bring with it guilt, shame, or moral judgments.

When I talk about intuitive eating, I am referring to the innate ability to listen to one's hunger and fullness signals. At its most basic level, it is knowing when to eat and when to stop. Intuitive eating also includes eating for well-being and pleasure and depends upon a level of body acceptance and self-trust.

Babies are born with the natural ability to signal when they are hungry and stop eating when they are full. Although children are born with the ability to eat intuitively, for a variety of reasons which I will discuss later, they start to lose this skill at about five years of age. This ability to tune in and pay attention to hunger and fullness is a gift, and I consider it your child's superpower. As parents, our job is to honor and protect that superpower, and in this book, I will show you how.

Rather than relying on external factors such as calories, macronutrients, time of day, or food rules, intuitive eating encourages tuning in and paying attention to the body's internal signals of hunger and satiety. Although this approach may seem odd or foreign in today's food culture, our ancestors fed themselves this way for thousands of years. Using external cues such as diet plans to determine how much to eat is a relatively new trend in our society that has been increasing over the past hundred years. Chemist Wilbur Olin Atwater discovered how to measure the calorie content of food in the late 1800s, but the concept of manipulating calorie intake for weight control was not popularized until the 1920s. *Diet and Health: With Key to the Calories*, written by physician Lulu Hunt Peters in 1918, was the first diet book to become a best seller. Peters herself used and promoted calorie counting as a weight-loss method.

Believe it or not, there was a time when people did not know their exact morning weight like their phone number or Social Security number. The bathroom scale did not arrive in homes until around 1910. Before this time, people did not weigh themselves regularly. Modern times have also provided an overabundance of food easily accessed with minimal effort. This radical shift in the availability of food combined with our desire for a culturally determined ideal body weight has led to the common practice of counting calories or measuring our food to determine how much to eat. We have been taught that we can't trust our bodies or our appetites, and our intake must be carefully controlled and restricted. The good news is that we actually have built-in physiological gauges that can guide us in eating the appropriate amount of food...if we pay attention. Many adults have unlearned this skill because we now use external factors to determine when to eat. However, when it comes to feeding our children, embracing and fostering their ability to eat intuitively will have many advantages for their health and long-term happiness.

I want to be very up-front about something. Intuitive eating is NOT a fad diet or novel weight-loss technique. It is a flexible, simple approach that is sustainable for a lifetime. You may even say that intuitive eating is the anti-diet. Intuitive eaters are not perfect, and we shouldn't expect ourselves or our children to become perfect intuitive eaters. It is not all-or-nothing or pass/fail; instead, it is an overall balanced pattern of eating and relating to food and our bodies.

In a sense, the concept of intuitive eating is very straightforward. However, it might not always feel natural to support the development of intuitive eating in your children through all the stages of growth. In Part III, I will discuss how to support and nurture your child's intuitive eating through the various developmental stages.

In addition to making logical sense, intuitive eating has research to support its benefits. Those that listen to their internal cues have less disordered eating behaviors, decreased odds of developing chronic dieting and binge eating, and are more likely to have lower body mass index. Intuitive eaters have also been found to have improved cholesterol markers and decreased cardiovascular risk. College women who scored high in intuitive eating were also more likely to be internally motivated to exercise for pleasure. Intuitive eaters are more likely to enjoy and take pleasure in their food and eating. And, what will come as an enormous relief to parents, intuitive eaters are *not* more likely to eat "junk" food. A review article exploring the results from 24 studies found that not only did participants have improved eating habits and body image, but they also exhibited less restriction, had increased body satisfaction, and showed improved psychological well-being. Even more impressive, many studies reported effects lasting up to three years. In a 2014 review article of 20 interventions that promoted eating by internal cues, the authors described one study in which 82 percent of the subjects had maintained intuitive eating and were able to identify hunger ten years after the intervention!

Intuitive eating achieves all three goals mentioned in Chapter 1 (see page 9). Along with well-being, health, body confidence, and self-trust, intuitive eating brings a decreased risk of chronic disease and a lower likelihood of disordered eating.

Since intuitive eating is based on hunger and satiety, it is essential to understand these concepts. Both are bodily processes that are regulated by complex chemical and hormonal cascades, but if we pay attention, we can tune into these sensations and honor them.

Chapter 3

Hunger and Satiety

B abies are born with an alarm system that triggers action when they are hungry and ready to eat. It's called crying! Most babies express other cues even before crying starts, and we search for these signs to know when to feed them. Babies, especially those who are breastfed, naturally stop when they are satisfied, then two or three hours later they start making signs that they are hungry again. If we try to feed them when they aren't hungry or force them to keep going when they are full, they often fuss or may even start crying again. We trust babies to alert us when they are hungry and, in general, parents are pretty good at picking up signs of hunger. But what exactly is hunger and why is it a beneficial sign?

What Is Hunger?

Hunger is the indication that it is time to eat. *The Oxford Dictionary* defines hunger as "a feeling of discomfort or weakness caused by lack of food, coupled with the desire to eat." Physical or physiological hunger occurs when the body biologically signals for more food. Mario Ciampolini, an Italian gastroenterologist at the University of Florence, and his colleagues identify two distinct hunger sensations: The first is called the "empty hollow sensation," when the stomach feels empty and you might experience hunger pangs or a growling stomach. This sensation explicitly indicates that the digestive system is ready to accept and digest food. The second is called "inanition," which is characterized by fatigue and light-headedness. Interestingly, both sensations correlate to a drop in blood sugar that determines an appropriate time to initiate eating.

There are multiple metabolic, hormonal, neurologic, and psychological processes that stimulate hunger and satiety. In the brain, the hypothalamus acts as the main control center for hunger and satiety and over fourteen hormones are involved. Ghrelin, a hormone that triggers hunger and motivates us to seek out food, is mainly produced in the stomach tissues. This hormone rises as it is closer to mealtime and falls after eating.

Ideally, we learn to pay attention to and respond most often to physical hunger. There are several benefits to this, including improved digestion and absorption of food. Ciampolini and his colleagues state that the desire to eat may occur in the absence of hunger, but hunger alone represents a state of physiological preparedness to digest. When we are physically hungry, it means that the body is physiologically ready to digest and absorb food. When this is the case, our metabolic processes are more efficient and effective.

A second health benefit to eating in response to physical hunger is improved insulin sensitivity and energy balance, which lead to weight regulation and can result in decreased inflammation and a lower risk of autoimmune disease.

Finally, food tastes much better when we are physically hungry. One of my favorite proverbs is "Hunger is the best sauce," meaning that when one is truly hungry, anything tastes good and excellent food tastes fantastic. One of the principles of intuitive eating is to derive pleasure and enjoyment from food. You can maximize pleasure from food by waiting for physical hunger before you eat. Seen this way, waiting to eat is not deprivation, but a way to derive more pleasure from your meal. When you experience physical hunger, your taste buds are open and ready!

However, eating is not always triggered by physiological hunger but other types of cues. Emotional hunger, or emotional eating, occurs when we develop habits or behaviors that link eating to our emotional states. Many adults and children have learned to eat when they are not hungry but, rather, bored, stressed, anxious, or sad. For example, it has become socially and culturally acceptable for women to manage the irritability and mood swings of premenstrual syndrome with the consumption of chocolate. It is also a common habit to use food to soothe a child or reward good behavior. This is not true hunger but a desire to eat outside of physical hunger.

Another type of hunger is a desire to eat that is triggered by external cues, such as time of day, seeing food, or behaviors like watching television, driving, or studying. We are often surrounded by food cues on television, on the radio, and in magazines, including where we work and as we drive. These food cues include images of food or people eating on billboards, magazines, television, and social media. There seems to be a constant bombardment of reminders to eat!

There is a scientific explanation for why seeing food suddenly makes us want to eat. The cephalic phase response is when our body becomes prepared for digestion by activating salivation and gastric juices, increasing heart rate, and releasing insulin. This physiological response is triggered by tasting, seeing, smelling, or even *thinking* about food! Research shows that there are differences in the strength of this response between individuals. Some people seem to have a stronger desire and motivation to eat after being exposed to these cues. Have you ever walked into a movie theater on a full stomach only to suddenly feel hungry after smelling the popcorn? Brian Wansink, a consumer researcher who has performed many studies on our eating habits, calls this the "see food" trap.

This cephalic phase response can also be conditioned or associated with other events. This psychological phenomenon is exemplified by the Pavlov's Dogs Study, in which the dogs in the experiment were trained to associate eating food to the ring of a bell. Upon the ringing of the bell, the dogs would start salivating in anticipation of eating, even though food was not physically present. The desire to eat popcorn upon walking into a movie theater is an example of conditioning. The first few times you arrive at a movie theater, smell and consume the popcorn, you create an association with popcorn and seeing a movie so that with time it becomes a habit to eat popcorn at the movies.

In *The Power of Habit*, Charles Duhigg breaks a habit down into three components: a cue, a routine, and a reward. This habit loop explains how certain events, such as sitting in front of the television or starting a study session, would become the "cue" that triggers the routine of eating. We are exposed to more food cues than ever before and we are responding to them by eating.

In the United States, the number of eating occasions has steadily increased over time. In 1977 children and adults ate an average of three times per day, and by 2006 that number had risen to six to seven eating occasions per day. This has resulted in a rise in daily calorie intake by about 443 calories and decreased time between meals with children eating about every three hours and adults every three-and-a-half hours. Given the results of these studies, it is likely that we are eating outside of physical hunger more often than before.

In our culture, mealtimes are usually set in our schedules and routines at daycare, school, and work. I remember watching my son's soccer game when he was around six years old. The game lasted only forty-five minutes, but the snack mom for the day handed out snacks before the game started, at halftime, and after the game was over. Another widespread practice is to eat several smaller meals throughout the day to prevent hunger. Because of this practice, many people have started to fear hunger and eat preemptively, completely ignoring hunger and fullness signals.

I want to emphasize that there is nothing shameful or wrong about non-hunger eating. We all do it from time to time (hello, Thanksgiving!). It is not a moral issue or a character defect. In some ways, it can be seen merely as an urge or a habit that has a real physiological and psychological basis. However, when non-hunger eating becomes the dominant cue for eating, it can lead to losing touch with true hunger and satiety. These habits can develop quickly and can lead to unwanted consequences. When we eat for emotional or external cues, we might be "hungry" in our minds, but not in our bodies. This means that our bodies may not be physically prepared to digest and absorb food. Eating outside of hunger can lead to indigestion, bloating, stomach pain, sluggishness, constipation, and diarrhea.

Although we all eat outside of hunger from time to time, it makes more sense to eat in response to physical hunger and stop when we feel satisfied. However, the process of satiety may be even more complex than hunger and less well understood.

What Is Satiety?

Knowing when to stop eating is a vital component of intuitive eating. Babies and young children are often sensitive to the internal cues that urge them to stop, sometimes after only a few bites, much to their parents' frustration. The sensation that often precedes stopping food intake is called "satiety."

Satiety refers to feeling satisfied with the amount of food that one has consumed. Certain hormones in the human body are associated with satiety, most notably cholecystokinin, peptide YY, insulin, leptin, and adiponectin. All of these hormones rise in response to satiety.

Sensing satiety is subtle and more challenging to recognize than physical hunger. Studies show that parents tend to be less responsive to satiety cues from their babies. There are several ways that we can determine if satiety has been reached. When satisfied, babies tend to turn their heads away, pull away from the breast, and cry if fed more. They are saying, "I have had enough." Just as we trust them to tell us when they are hungry, we must trust them when they indicate to us or tell us they have had enough. When you approach fullness, the taste of food actually changes and becomes less delicious. Your rate of eating may slow down, and you may find yourself distracted by something else. When other things become more attractive than food, it is a sign that you or your child has had enough.

Children maintain this skill of being in tune with their hunger and satiety as they grow. Toddlers are especially good at this, and it creates immense distress for parents. Toddlers love to play and explore their world. In fact, that is their number-one job. Many of them can't be bothered to sit and eat if they are not hungry. Some days it seems like they hardly have an appetite, and other days they seem insatiable. This is completely normal. I encourage parents to support this natural intuition. As long as your child is a developmentally normal child and growing on their growth curve, do not worry about these normal behaviors. When children learn to eat past fullness, they can start to develop unhealthy habits.

Although hunger and satiety are easy concepts to understand, they are not black and white. Just as there are genes that account for fixed physical traits such as eye color and height, genetic components may also influence behavioral characteristics, including our eating behaviors. The speed of eating, how much one eats, or how much interest and enjoyment a person takes in food is rooted in our genes. This is evident even in newborns that exhibit different feeding cues and behaviors.

I would call myself a food lover and, apparently, this has been true since early childhood. According to my grandmother, one afternoon when I was a toddler, as my aunt was sitting at the table eating her lunch, I snuck by and with my little toddler hands swiped a large piece of food off of her plate, running away and happily announcing "Rico!" which means "delicious" in Spanish. My older son has inherited my eating gusto. He takes a very high interest in food and would even dance in his high chair when something was particularly delicious to him. My younger son can appreciate food and does enjoy it, but definitely not to the same level. He is also more likely to wait to eat until he is physically hungry, and he does not enjoy eating in the absence of hunger. He likes to finish his meals quickly so he can do other things, while my older son and I linger at the table, taking distinct pleasure in our meals. Maybe you see differences like this in your children and family members, but my point here is that these differences are normal, to be expected, and nothing to worry about. It's really the eating habits that we instill in our children by honoring their hunger and satiety cues that make the difference in their long-term health.

How Pleasure and Food Connect

In our culture, delicious food is often labeled "sinful," "decadent," or as a "guilty" pleasure. We have become one of the most health-conscious countries in the world, but we also derive the least satisfaction from our food. This is likely because we have created excessive rules around our eating and have become accustomed to labeling foods as "good" or "bad." Research shows that the more health conscious a person is, the less likely they are to derive pleasure from their food and the less likely they are to be intuitive eaters. Orthorexia nervosa, also known as orthorexia, is a form of disordered eating that has been gaining more attention in recent years. People that suffer from this disorder become obsessed with a healthy diet to the point that it begins to interrupt their life and well-being. They may avoid eating out and going to social functions, and they become fearful of more and more foods. Restrained eaters are those who are purposely restricting their dietary intake to lose weight or maintain weight loss. Unrestrained eaters, on the other hand, are not bound by food rules or diets. Intuitive eaters are naturally unrestrained eaters. They seek enjoyable nourishment when they are physically hungry. Ironically, although restrained eaters aim to reduce their calorie intake, they actually end up consuming more calories than they intend because the restriction often leads to binge eating and emotional eating. They also experience higher levels of guilt after eating and are more likely to be attracted to high-calorie foods.

When we make eating choices from a place of dietary restraint, it limits the pleasure we derive from our food. Pleasure and enjoyment come through all the senses: our vision, our smell, and our taste. It is also felt inside the body. Intuitive eaters tune into their bodies and know which foods lead to feeling good and which cause feelings and sensations that they do not enjoy. Although a plate of salty, greasy fries might taste good in the mouth, it may not feel good in the body, and an intuitive eater can make decisions based on these past learned experiences. An intuitive eater can receive and interpret the body's feedback and use it to determine their eating decisions.

Pleasure is not wrong or sinful. We deserve joy in life, and it is not just okay, but beneficial to derive pleasure from our food. One intriguing study found that eating a highly desired food item decreased cravings for more food. This means that when we eat what we really enjoy, we gain pleasure and satisfaction, and our desire to keep eating decreases, making it easier to eat within hunger and satiety.

Chapter 4

Body Acceptance

Concern over your weight may increase your worry for your children and influence how you feed them. Body size obsession, dissatisfaction with body size, and dieting behavior can be passed down through generations. I have observed this in my practice, among my friends and family members, and in my own personal life.

I grew up watching my mother complain about her body, express disgust and frustration with her size and shape, and diet in some extreme ways. It is therefore no surprise that I started dieting at age nine. My mom and I often dieted (and "cheated" on our diets) together. I remember accompanying her and her friend to a nearby town, where they would see a weight-loss specialist to get diet pills. Ironically, I loved these trips because on the way home we would stop for ice cream. I was way too young at the time to appreciate the irony of that monthly ritual.

In my family, body fat was frequently criticized and viewed as undesirable, and being dissatisfied with one's own body was accepted and normalized. In 1984, Dr. Judith Rodin, then a research psychologist and professor at Yale University, named this "normative discontent," which basically means that it is "normal" to be dissatisfied with the appearance of one's body. It is prevalent in many families, especially in American culture.

Fear and anxiety over weight naturally lead to control over food and eating. To truly embrace intuitive eating and develop a healthy relationship with food, it is necessary to let go of the need to rigidly control weight.

It's commonly thought that to change or improve, a person should be unsatisfied, unhappy, or perhaps even loathe the part of themselves they wish to change. However, one study found that body esteem was the only predictor of weight maintenance at a one-year follow-up. This means that respecting and accepting your body (rather than hating it) is more likely to lead to healthy behaviors that help regulate body weight.

If you have suffered from disordered eating, dieting, and poor body image, you are not alone. An Ipsos national poll in 2018 found that 79 percent of Americans felt unhappy with the appearance of their body, and according to a 2011 Gallup poll, 30 percent of American adults have attempted weight loss between three and ten times in their lives.

Women are more likely to diet than men, and they are also likely to influence their children through this behavior. At least 75 percent of women have attempted to lose weight in their lifetimes. Girls are starting to diet at younger and younger ages. One study found that the desire for thinness for little girls emerged at the shockingly young age of six. This was more likely to be the case when these girls' mothers were themselves dissatisfied with their bodies. Another study found that between 34 to 65 percent of five-year-old girls already had beliefs about dieting. One study found that if mothers were dieting, their daughters were nearly three times more likely to start dieting before age eleven. Similarly, another study revealed that a mother's worry about her own weight was predictive of body dissatisfaction and dieting in her daughters and sons five years later. The more mothers worried about their weight, the higher the odds that their daughters would diet even if the daughters themselves were not overweight.

Poor body image in mothers may also lead to some unexpected consequences. Mothers with poor body image are less likely to initiate breastfeeding due to embarrassment or concern about how breastfeeding may impact their body.

Dieting is incompatible with intuitive eating. Dieting imposes rules that dictate when, what, and how much to eat. This leads to either ignoring hunger signals and undereating or dismissing fullness and overeating because consuming a certain amount is part of "the plan." This reliance on external cues to determine when and how much to eat teaches new habits that are in opposition to eating intuitively. When we are dieting, we are not eating intuitively.

Our own dissatisfaction with our bodies makes it difficult to teach intuitive eating to our children because we are often not modeling the foundational principles of this practice. Our own fear of being "fat" can be transferred to the way we feed our children or talk about weight and eating. Mothers who are worried about their own weight tend to worry more about their children's weight. If we perceive that our children overeat or desire foods that we believe are "fattening," this can lead us to consciously or subconsciously restrict certain foods to "protect" our children. Our fear can lead us to become very controlling and can interfere with supporting intuitive eating. Research shows that mothers who eat intuitively are less likely to try to control their children's intake. So, the best way for your children to become intuitive eaters is to let go of dieting and model intuitive eating instead.

Health at Every Size

The most common argument for dieting is that overweight or obese people will not be healthy unless they diet and lose weight. One recurrent popular news story is that we are living in an obesity epidemic that is slowly killing us and shortening our life spans. News stories show pictures of overweight adults and kids eating hamburgers and ice cream. Some of us shake our heads, and others feel ashamed. I have to admit, early in my career, I would share these statistics with families often. I thought that maybe if people were aware of the "problem," it would help them develop the motivation to make healthy lifestyle changes.

Contrary to popular belief, fear is not a strong motivator for long-term behavior change. In fact, the fearmongering surrounding weight and body size can actually cause harm. Millions of people in the United States go on a diet every year. And millions of people lose weight only to gain it back again. They then feel like failures, and, demoralized, perhaps they try something even more drastic the next time, quickly losing and regaining the weight for several weight cycles. Even worse, they may begin to feel that they are worthless failures because they just can't seem to keep the weight off. They may avoid social and family events because of their size or weight and eventually, they may just give up, feeling like a healthy weight just isn't possible for them. Socially, weight stigma, discrimination, and bias can be painful and isolating, but medically it can be dangerous. Diagnoses can be delayed or missed because symptoms are either attributed to weight or because a person might seem protected from a certain disease and not tested due to their naturally lean size. Additionally, many larger people may put off going to a doctor because they fear the scale or judgment from their health-care provider. One study found that as many as one-third of women have avoided or delayed health care because they had gained weight, feared that they would be told to lose weight, or did not want to get weighed.

If fear is not the best motivator for long-term healthy behavior change, what is? I believe that it is love, compassion, and self-acceptance. Health at Every Size removes the focus from weight and body size and instead places it on health and well-being. This approach to eating emphasizes that anybody can pursue healthy behaviors *regardless* of their size or weight. I love this philosophy because it places controllable and actionable behaviors as the means to achieve well-being, rather than setting an arbitrary number that may be beyond a person's control as the end goal. Linda Bacon, author of the books *Health at Every Size* and *Body Respect*, breaks HAES down into three main concepts: compassionate self-care, respect, and critical awareness. Compassionate self-care refers to eating intuitively and in a way that is pleasurable and aligned with the body, as well as finding joy and pleasure in movement. Respect means celebrating body diversity and honoring individual differences in every aspect. Critical awareness encourages valuing our own lived experiences and body knowledge as well as challenging cultural and scientific assumptions.

The Association for Size Diversity and Health summarizes the Health at Every Size principles beautifully. These principles can be found on the association's website and are intended to help individuals who are looking for a non-diet approach to health and also professionals who aim to support patients and clients in this paradigm. These five principles are:

1. **Weight inclusivity:** Accept and respect the inherent diversity of body shapes and sizes and reject the idealizing or pathologizing of specific weights.

2. **Health enhancement:** Support health policies that improve and equalize access to information and services, and personal practices that improve human well-being, including attention to individual physical, economic, social, spiritual, emotional, and other needs.

3. **Respectful care:** Acknowledge our biases, and work to end weight discrimination, weight stigma, and weight bias. Provide information and services from an understanding that socioeconomic status, race, gender, sexual orientation, age, and other identities impact weight stigma, and support environments that address these inequities.

4. **Eating for well-being:** Promote flexible, individualized eating based on hunger, satiety, nutritional needs, and pleasure rather than on any externally regulated eating plan focused on weight control.

5. **Life-enhancing movement:** Support physical activities that allow people of all sizes, abilities, and interests to engage in enjoyable movements, to the degree that they choose.

The Health at Every Size movement has been misinterpreted as the belief that everybody is healthy regardless of their size or weight. This is not the intent or philosophy of HAES. But I do want to take this opportunity to clarify that having a certain body weight neither dooms you to poor health nor makes you immune from disease. The point is that taking weight and body size out of the end goal and, instead, developing habits and behaviors that promote health and well-being is actually *more* health-promoting than merely trying to lose weight (over and over again). I believe that HAES is for *everyone*. Even though we tend to value thinness in our current society, there is a large percentage of thin people who are unhappy with their size or shape. This may be especially true for men who would like to be larger and more muscular. Just like we all don't have the same eye color and aren't the same height, we aren't all going to be the same weight and clothing size.

Health at Every Size is not a popular philosophy among those in the health movement. It is not going to help sell diet books or weight-loss programs. Many believe that if we don't scare people about their weight or health, they won't try to do anything to change their health status. However, I believe that the opposite is true. When we stop pressuring people to reach a certain number or percentage, they are instead able to focus on habits and behaviors that promote health and well-being, bring them authentic joy, and fit into a sustainable lifestyle.

When we start to focus instead on eating, moving, and living for health and joy rather than for size and weight, something magical happens. We feel immense freedom, happiness, and acceptance. We make better choices that align with our values and our genetic makeup.

I recommend approaching weight in children consistent with the principles of HAES. Instead of emphasizing weight, adopt healthy habits and behaviors. If a child is thriving, eating wholesome foods, sleeping well, and free of chronic conditions, then they are likely operating at their genetic potential, regardless of their size.

Several studies have found that applying the principles of HAES is associated with improved self-esteem and body image, health behaviors such as improved dietary quality, increased physical activity, and even physiological measures such as decreased blood pressure and cholesterol. With HAES, people are more likely to reduce their intake of processed foods and increase their intake of fruits and vegetables. Because intuitive eating is a component of HAES, women who learn and implement HAES principles are more likely to learn to eat intuitively and are also more likely to have improved body esteem and less dieting behaviors compared to women who diet.

Although HAES is a broader philosophy that goes beyond just eating intuitively, it is a way of thinking that will support intuitive eating because it removes the pressure to diet to achieve a specific body size. It emphasizes health and joy, which are ultimately more helpful in gauging whether you and your family are on track with your eating and nutrition choices.

HAES is still not the conventional medical model and may not be for a while. It is likely that body weight will continue to be the focus for some years to come.

Feeding Practices vs. Intuitive Eating

Eighty-five percent of all parents actually try to get their children to eat more. This is usually with good intentions. However, it often creates the opposite result. Children pressured to eat actually avoid food more, eat *fewer* fruits and vegetables, and consume more processed foods. For these children, eating is no longer pleasurable and can become a stressful daily experience, leading to even more avoidance.

Similarly, restricting food quantity or certain types of foods to control a child's weight tends to augment that child's desire to seek food, and, ironically, can lead to more weight gain. They may develop behaviors such as hoarding, sneaking food, and bingeing, and they are more likely to engage in unhealthy and extreme weight control practices in the future. Forced restriction causes a feeling of scarcity, which can trigger these behaviors.

These same behaviors may also be present in children who experience food scarcity from neglect or poverty.

Emotional feeding is when parents give food to their children in an attempt to influence their behavior or change their emotional state. Children who are fed this way are more likely to become emotional eaters. And although there are possible genetic differences in susceptibility to emotional eating, a twin study showed that when it comes to emotional eating, environmental influence is more predictive than genetics. Emotional eating is not intuitive eating, and it is a habit that can lead to adverse health consequences. The practice of using food as a reward or as a soothing technique is associated with obesity in children. Mothers who feed their children for emotional reasons are more likely to introduce juice and solids at an early age and breastfeed their children for a shorter duration. The more children learn to eat for a feeling of reward or to soothe negative emotions, the more out of tune they will become with their natural hunger and satiety signals. The bottom line is that emotional eating is taught. The best way to avoid promoting this habit in your child is to avoid using food as a reward or punishment.

Parents and caregivers who pressure children to eat more or restrict their intake or selection of foods often do so out of concern over their child's weight. These weight concerns stem from a variety of sources. However, in my experience, they are unfounded. I spend a lot of time reassuring parents that their child is at a normal, healthy weight. Understanding growth charts and the normal growth patterns of children can help reassure you that your child is thriving.

Growth Curves Explained

When parents come to me concerned about their child's growth, the first thing I do is review their growth charts. Honestly, the majority of the time, I reassure parents. Although there are genetic, metabolic, and medical conditions that can lead to inappropriate growth, this is rare, and if a child is otherwise thriving and developing normally, their weight is not usually a problem.

Growth charts were first developed in the late eighteenth century by Count Philibert de Montbeillard, but pediatricians have been using them in the United States since the 1970s. For newborns to children age of three, we monitor weight (usually in pounds), length (usually in inches), head circumference, and weight-for-length. Weight-for-length is used to assess body mass and appropriate weight gain for the length of a child. In a weight-for-length chart, the length is plotted on the x-axis and the weight on the y-axis. After age two we also monitor body mass index (BMI), a number calculated by dividing body weight by height, usually weight divided by height squared. BMI is meant to be a rough estimate of body fat. BMI is not a precise measurement and is calculated the same way for everyone, regardless of age or gender. In adults over the age of eighteen, the recommended BMI range is 18.5 to 25, with 25 to 30 classified as overweight and over 30 classified as obese. In children, instead of using specific number cutoffs, we use percentiles to determine risk categories. A typical child will fall between 5th and 85th percentiles. Overweight is considered 85th to 95th percentile, obese is over 95th percentile, and underweight is less than the 5th percentile.

Boys and girls have separate growth charts stratified by age. Growth curves are based on population data and organized into percentiles with age of the child (months or years of age) on the x-axis and either weight, height, head circumference, or BMI on the y-axis. In the United States, many health-care providers use the World Health Organization (WHO) growth charts, which were created using the data of healthy, typically developing, breastfed children from six different countries to set standards for what is believed to be healthy growth. Another set of growth charts are the Centers for Disease Control and Prevention (CDC) growth charts that were created using data on American children that has been collected since the 1960s. The WHO charts are typically used in the first two years of life and the CDC growth charts are used from age two through twenty.

What does a data point on a growth chart represent? If you were to find one hundred two-month-old babies, put them in the same room, and weigh and measure them, they would invariably be all different weights and heights. When these data are plotted on a curve, it creates what is called a "normal curve" or a "bell curve." The center of the curve is where the majority of the children lie, but there will likely be some kids that are much bigger or much smaller. The middle of the curve is the fiftieth percentile and represents both the median and the mean of the weight or the length (or height) of the child. This means that approximately half of children will be above this and half will be below, and the distance away from the center delineates percentiles. Most children will fall within the chart for their weight, height, and head circumference, but sometimes if they are very tall, heavy, or have large heads, they may be "greater than the 97th percentile," or if they are very small they may be "less than the 3rd percentile."

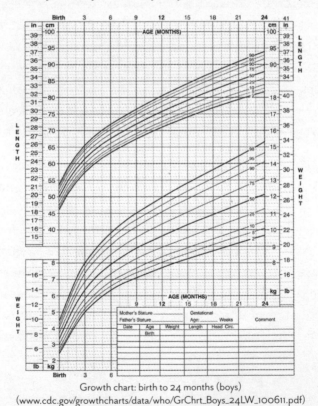

Growth chart: birth to 24 months (boys)
(www.cdc.gov/growthcharts/data/who/GrChrt_Boys_24LW_100611.pdf)

a parent's guide to intuitive eating

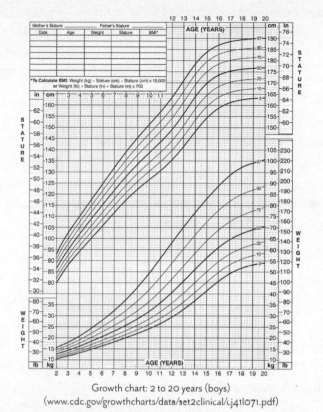

Growth chart: 2 to 20 years (boys)
(www.cdc.gov/growthcharts/data/set2clinical/cj41l071.pdf)

Published by the CDC; sourced from WHO child growth standards

What does this mean for your child? Just as adults come in all shapes and sizes, so do kids. When your health-care provider monitors the growth charts, they are looking for trends over time. This is why it is crucial to have multiple points of data on the growth curve.

The percentile for your child is not a grade or a pass/fail. Additionally, a higher percentile is not necessarily better or worse than a lower percentile. Not all children are going to fall at the 75th percentile. If your child has always been at the 10th percentile for their weight and height and they are developing normally and thriving, this is likely where their genetics has destined them to be. When I interpret growth curves, I determine if children are roughly following their percentile lines over time. If they start falling down in percentiles, their curve flattens over time, or they show sharp increases, that is when I get concerned. There are a few exceptions to this. Changes can occur around puberty that lead to a sudden surge in growth, but once puberty is complete, growth decelerates, and their curve flattens. Babies tend to reach what we call their "true curve" between nine and fifteen months. We call it this because in the beginning, babies, especially breastfed babies, can appear larger than what they will ultimately be. Breast milk can create deliciously plump babies, and this is actually protective of later obesity, but they won't necessarily always stay at such a high percentile. Between nine and fifteen months, many babies also became mobile and growth velocity for weight slows down a bit so they may become leaner in appearance. This is all normal.

I often use growth charts to reassure parents who are concerned that their toddler isn't eating enough, but sometimes growth charts can create anxiety if they are misunderstood. Parents will express concern, for instance, when they see that their typically developing, thriving child is tracking along the 25th percentile. They worry that they have a "small child" and ask if there is something that they need to do to help him/her grow better. If their child is tracking well along their curves and is healthy and vigorous, I reassure them that they should continue to do precisely what they have been doing because it is working great! When it comes to size, our height and weight have strong genetic influences. Studies of identical twins separated at birth found that genetics account for 70 percent of the determinants of body mass index.

My job as a pediatrician is to optimize nutrition and well-being so that children are free to grow and develop to their genetic potential. What I want you to remember is that your child has their own genetic instructions for what their ultimate height and body type will be.

Body Type Differences

The Lean Child

Some children are naturally lean. As long as they are following their growth curves and not flattening out or falling off their growth curve and they are happy and developing well, there is no reason for concern. Often one or both parents remember being very lean as children and might still be in adulthood. They might use words like "skinny" or "lanky" to describe how they were when they were children. However, parents of lean children can fall into two traps. The first is the lean person bias. This is the assumption that just because a child is lean they can and should eat "whatever they want because at least they're eating!" These parents are concerned that if the child is not eating Pop-Tarts and mac and cheese all the time, they will literally wither away.

The second trap is thinking that just because the child is lean, they are not at risk of chronic disease later in life. This is the opposite of how we feel about larger people and their increased risk of lifestyle-related chronic disease. Larger people are considered unhealthy until proven otherwise and lean people tend to get a free pass because we assume they are healthy because they are slim.

No matter what kind of body type a child has, I still stick with the same recommendations for most children. Establish healthy habits and center your family's meals around fruits, vegetables, whole grains, beans, and nuts and seeds. Promote intuitive eating. Don't forget about your responsibility to provide the food and routines, and your child's autonomy to decide how much he or she wants to eat. Even if a person is lean on the outside, the INSIDE is relevant too. We get our insides healthy and disease-resistant by eating a health-promoting diet and living a healthy lifestyle.

Just like parents with larger children, parents with lean children may get unsolicited comments from strangers, family members, or health professionals who are not well-trained on interpreting growth charts. If you feel that you are getting undue pressure from your physician, you may consider getting a second opinion from a pediatrician who is familiar with growth trends. If you do choose to see another physician, ensure that they have access to all of your child's growth charts and growth and developmental history.

Tips for supporting your naturally lean child:

- Continue to offer health-promoting meals and snacks on a regular schedule.

- Avoid falling into the trap of becoming a short-order cook or giving in to every request for preferred foods because you are worried your child is too small.

- Never force them to eat; respect their satiety cues.

- Avoid making comments, teasing, or creating nicknames about their size or weight. This can be just as hurtful as it is for larger children and can create self-consciousness.

- Stand your ground and be an advocate for your child when you encounter comments from strangers and family members.

These changes take time, especially if your family is only starting to learn the principles of intuitive eating and emphasizing health-promoting foods. There will be ups and downs as you continue on this journey, but it will get easier.

I am also aware that because we are such a weight-focused society, you may hear the opposite message from well-meaning friends, family members, and even medical professionals who are not familiar with or advocates of Health at Every Size. I am also very aware of the shaming that occurs to parents of larger children. It breaks my heart. It may be difficult to stand your ground and feel confident in your choices when you encounter comments and societal messages like this, but I wholeheartedly believe that dieting and restriction are not the answer to raising healthy and happy children. Be an advocate for your child and your conviction that their size and weight is not an indicator of their health and well-being. However, you may still feel anxiety or sadness. If you are struggling, seek support or professional help for yourself.

The Large Child

In pediatrics, we define overweight as a body mass index (BMI) greater than 85th percentile and obesity as a BMI greater than 95th percentile. Despite these numbers and current guidelines, in my practice, I look at the whole picture. Even for kids whose BMI is greater than 85th percentile, if they are also tall, active, eat a healthy diet, and have healthy lifestyle habits, I do not get concerned, especially if they have always been of a larger size. The most important thing to me is that they have healthy long-term habits. Some people are going to be larger than others. However, if the BMI is rising sharply, I start to dig deeper to see if other factors may be contributing to excess weight gain.

My main plea to parents is to not make a big deal over the size of your child's body. If you are concerned, talk to your pediatrician in private, but don't make a habit of focusing so much on the size or shape of your child's body. Instead, spend your time discussing *healthy habits* and health-promoting foods and having a healthy relationship with food and eating. If you have suffered from overweight, obesity, or an eating disorder, you may panic if you have a larger child. If you are feeling a lot of anxiety and struggling with this, it may be worth seeing a therapist. Overfocus on body size and eating-disorder tendencies tend to get passed down, and it can lead to a lifelong struggle for your child.

If your child has been diagnosed as overweight or obese, my biggest tip is to adopt the principles of intuitive eating. Start emphasizing healthy habits and let the body do what it will. Unless there is a medical problem that necessitates weight loss, there is no need to focus on weight loss or reaching a specific body size or BMI. Size and body fat is only one determinant of health, and it is not even the most important one. The key then is to *continue* those habits for the long-term, and they will pay off.

Tips for supporting your large child:

- Shift your focus from body size or shape to health and well-being. Believe that your child is and can be healthy NOW, regardless of their size. Review the principles of Health at Every Size and focus on appreciating your child for all the beautiful qualities that they have.

- Practice intuitive eating and body confidence yourself. Be a role model for healthy habits and appreciate your body.

- Adopt a health-promoting diet for the entire family. Do not make a special diet just for the child that struggles with weight.

- Help your child learn to tune into hunger and satiety. Be patient. This takes time.

- Get your child active in a sport or after-school physical activity that they enjoy and find pleasurable.

- Be a role model and continue to improve your healthy eating and exercise habits right along with your child.

- Do not single out your child or try to shame them or guilt them into changing their eating habits.

- If you suspect your child is a chronic overeater and is having problems with binge eating or hiding food, model the principles of intuitive eating, make sure you are not restricting food, and seek out a therapist that specializes in eating disorders.

- Be patient, do your best, and let go of the outcome.

How to Foster a Healthy Body Image in Your Children

To support healthy body image in our children, we must be mindful of what we say and what messages we convey in our home environment. Although we do not have absolute control over everything that our child sees or hears, there are ways that we can send positive ideas about bodies to our children that will help counteract what they encounter out in the world.

What You Say Matters

Many of us criticize our bodies in front of our children. "Fat talk," or putting down our weight and shape, is correlated with and may even be a cause of body dissatisfaction, especially among girls and women. Before I changed my habits in this area, I would say things like, "Ugh, I feel so fat!" or "My butt is just so big!" usually with disgust in my voice and face. I was surprised to hear my six-year-old mirror this language about his own body, not knowing he had been paying attention.

Language around body dissatisfaction is so pervasive that you may not even realize that you do it. Discussing body parts that you are unhappy with or the need to lose weight, "get in shape," or "slim down" are all ways of saying that you want to lose weight. No matter how you say it, if you are talking about being unhappy about the size or shape of your body, you convey to your child that it is something that you value for yourself and perhaps for them as well. However, language can also center around food, from discussing calorie content to how "fattening" a particular food is. My point here is that how we talk about our own bodies impacts our children. It can also create a negative feedback cycle for the person engaging in language about body dissatisfaction.

Reflections on Baby Fat

Human babies are born with the highest percentage of body fat of all mammals, with 10 to 15 percent body fat at birth. But in the next few months, they put on even more fat, with baby girls getting up to around 30 percent body fat after four-and-a-half months. This body fat gives human babies a survival advantage that has paid off for the human species. I have the privilege of seeing healthy, beautiful babies in my office every day. They have rolls upon rolls, double chins, no neck, and cellulite on their bare bottoms. There is nothing more delightful than bringing these warm, sweet-smelling babies into a warm embrace and squeezing their pillowy marshmallowy softness. Who doesn't love a chubby baby?

It's interesting that fat transitions so drastically from a desired and celebrated attribute to something that is so hated and despised. When we see fat on babies, we don't view it as disgusting or shameful, but when we see it on ourselves, we attribute it to a deep character flaw or a moral failing. It's just fat! Even though we tend to demonize fat, it actually serves many vital purposes in our body. In her book *The Secret Life of Fat*, author Sylvia Tara reveals all the fascinating functions of fat. Dr. Tara informs us that fat is "involved in the management of our energy stores, thermal regulation, keeping our cells intact, and, surprisingly, in sending signals within our bodies." Body fat is essential for reproduction. For females, it's critical to have a minimum amount of body fat in order to ovulate, menstruate, and carry a baby. Maybe fat doesn't seem so cute on adults in our current society, but it really is a necessary body organ. Even if you can't love it, appreciate that our bodies need it to function properly.

The way that we talk to our children about *their* eating and bodies is also important. Mothers of obese children are more likely to use harsh words or tone of voice when attempting to control their food intake. Sometimes mothers may even try to shame their children into eating less. In some families, parents or siblings may tease children about their bodies. It may seem innocent and something that is common and pervasive but can lead to strong psychological effects. A fifteen-year longitudinal study found that women who were teased about their weight by family and peers during adolescence had a higher BMI and adverse eating outcomes such as poor body image, emotional eating, unhealthy weight control methods, and binge eating fifteen years later. Body weight may be one of the most common reasons young people are teased and bullied. We may not be able to control what happens outside the home, but in our homes, we can choose to refrain from teasing children about their weight. This is just as important for lean children. Nobody should be teased about their body size or shape.

Media Exposure

It is well known that exposure to media has many effects on our thoughts and behaviors. Many people believe that they are above the effects of advertising, but children are particularly susceptible and easily influenced by marketing. Food companies specifically target advertising spots during children's television to market breakfast cereals and snack foods. Studies find that children who watch more TV have an increased preference for energy-dense foods, sweet beverages, and snacking, and eat less fruits and vegetables. And children tend to then influence their parents on what to purchase. The cephalic phase response (page 17) comes into play here. When children see ads for food, it can trigger false hunger and increase eating.

Children who eat in front of the television are more likely to be distracted and less in touch with their satiety signals. Children consume 24 percent more calories when watching TV. Food marketing also appears in magazines and social media, and it has become so pervasive that it is almost impossible to escape. Social media influencers are now paid to market products to children who often can't tell that it is an ad. In a study on social media influencer marketing, it was found that these influencer ads led to an overall higher intake of food and unhealthy snacks. Unfortunately, viewing influencers with healthy snacks did not significantly increase consumption of fruits and vegetables.

What might be even more subtle is the influence of media on our perceptions of ideal body size. It can also transmit ideas about dieting and social acceptance. Even if you do a great job of promoting healthy body image and body acceptance at home, the media will have repeated messages about weight loss and other body-focused themes. Young adults, both male and female, who spend more time on social media are more likely to have disordered eating. Social media can be particularly influential to kids and teens and can lower body esteem very quickly, especially for young women.

My recommendations on media exposure may seem extreme and radical, but my feeling is that the influence of media on young minds is so strong that it is our responsibility to make sure our children are not overexposed to these messages before they are prepared to process them. In this day and age, media exposure is determined by screen time. "Screen time" is time spent on any device with a screen, such as televisions, computers, video game consoles, smartphones, or tablets.

1. Under two. Do not expose children younger than two years old to screen time. The American Academy of Pediatrics guidelines state that children under two not partake in screen time at all. Besides the influence it can have on children, it can also interfere with speech development.

2. Over two. Allow children over two an hour of supervised screen time per day. Avoid television with advertising if possible.

3. Magazines. Avoid subscribing to magazines that have body-focused, weight loss, or dieting themes. These magazines tend to recirculate the same stories about weight loss over and over again, and promote a thin ideal. If you must purchase these types of magazines, consider getting a digital-only subscription or keeping them out of view of your children so that only you see them.

4. Social Media. Do not allow your children to have social media accounts until they are old enough. Many social media accounts prohibit children younger than thirteen from having accounts because the Children's Online Privacy Protection Act of 1998, a United States Federal law, restricts the collection of data and marketing to children under the age of thirteen. Children younger than a certain age will also be more susceptible to online dangers. There are many disadvantages to social media. My sons are currently nine and fourteen years old and do not have phones or social media accounts. I know that times are different now but being on social media is definitely not necessary. You will have to find what works for your family. Once your child does create a social media account, ensure that they have adequate security settings, discuss safe and unsafe practices, and check their use frequently. Also talk to your child about the reality that not everything they see online is real.

5. Advertisements. Openly discuss advertisements and marketing to children so that they understand and critically evaluate what they see. This will not make them immune to advertising, but it will at least allow them to develop a healthy skepticism and critical thinking.

Body Image Over Time

By age six, children understand the concept of dieting. Children at this age are very impressionable and will model what you do. It is especially critical at this age and beyond that you practice your own intuitive eating and avoid making disparaging remarks about your own body or anybody else's. Show your child that all bodies are good bodies, and it is our habits and behaviors that help us stay healthy and happy.

Many girls will start dieting in childhood around the time of puberty. At puberty, not only do children's bodies change in dramatic ways, but they also begin to care more about their appearance and what other people think about them. This can be a dangerous combination, especially if they have absorbed the message that being thinner or more muscular is better. Some personality types may be more susceptible to these messages, but you can also provide a positive influence to protect your child from falling into the dieting and weight-obsessed culture.

How to promote a healthy body image in your children:

1. **Be a role model for positive body image.** Practice intuitive eating rather than dieting or restrictive eating practices.

2. **Be aware of your own talk.** Sometimes we may start focusing on our personal appearances without even realizing it. If you notice yourself being critical of your own or another's appearance, keep it in check to avoid sending this message to your child.

3. **Avoid teasing children.** This includes creating nicknames that are focused on size or weight. This is more common in some families and cultures. Even if it seems cute, it can be triggering for some children.

4. **Keep the lines of communication open.** Talk to your child about worries or concerns they may have about their body. Don't tiptoe around the normal biological changes that occur during childhood and puberty. Once your child's body starts changing (or even before!) and your child expresses concerns or curiosity about their body, talk to them about how they feel and ask if they have questions or concerns about the changes they are experiencing.

5. **Reassure your child that body size and weight fluctuate over a lifetime.** This is a healthy and natural phenomenon. Humans are designed to grow and adapt and change over time. This is especially true at certain milestones in life, such as puberty and pregnancy.

6. **Remind your child that they have inherent worth and are loved regardless of their body size, shape, or weight, or any other physical characteristic.** Talk to them about positive relationships and how to choose friends who also value them for who they are.

7. **Don't promote dieting or other restrictive practices to change the appearance of their body.** Help your child focus on health and function rather than appearance, and continue to encourage a health-promoting and intuitive way of eating rather than restriction or deprivation. Empower them to be in control of their health and well-being by making choices that promote balance and joy. Teach them about Health at Every Size and how to continue health-promoting habits that feel good to them.

8. **Talk about food in terms of health and pleasure, not in terms of calories.** Discuss how foods benefit our health and help us feel good rather than how they help us lose weight or prevent weight gain.

9. **Focus on qualities other than appearance.** Although children become more focused on appearance around adolescence, help them build their self-confidence and remember all of the other traits and qualities that they have and the many ways they can build and develop them.

10. **Teach your kids to be critical of media images and our dieting culture.** Openly talk about advertisements, marketing campaigns, or language that promote a certain body ideal. Educate them about social media images and the illusion of perfection that can be created through various forms of digital manipulation. Help them see how weight and size bias can impact advertisements and how it makes people feel. Show respect and appreciation for all body types.

The Reality of Disordered Eating

Even for those children whose parents support intuitive eating, a percentage of children will still eventually develop disordered eating or an eating disorder. It's not your fault. Do the best you can and let go of the outcome after that. Remember that our eating behaviors are complex and made up of many components. As parents, we simply do not have 100 percent control. Learn the concepts of intuitive eating and adapt them to your family and personal situation. I commend you for the courage to learn these techniques so that you can do the best you can for your children.

It has taken me some time, patience, self-acceptance, and persistence to break the patterns of dieting, binge eating, and discomfort with my own body. Being aware of these patterns and beliefs is imperative to become deliberate in your efforts to support and foster intuitive eating in your little ones. If you feel trapped by cycles of negative body image and recurrent dieting and want to break free, here are some tips for you:

1. Accept yourself as you are this very moment. Many people spend years living in a state of pause because they put off doing the things they want to do until they arrive at a magical weight or clothing size. Accepting yourself as you are does not mean you can't take measures to improve your health or well-being, but it does mean moving on and doing the things that bring you joy and authentic pleasure. Self-acceptance does not mean you have to love every part of your body, it just means you accept where you are at the present moment.

2. Stop dieting. Dieting can be addictive and create a repetitive pattern of hope, excitement, disappointment, and despair over and over again. As I have said before, dieting is incompatible with intuitive eating and will prohibit you from learning the skills of honoring your hunger and satiety. Not dieting can cause significant anxiety and sadness initially, but it gets easier over time, especially as you experience the freedom that comes with eating without restrictive food rules.

3. Get rid of your scale. Consider not weighing yourself even if it's just for a short break. The number on the scale should not determine your happiness or self-worth. A better way to self-monitor is to tune in and pay attention to how your body feels on a day-to-day basis and how you feel in your clothes.

4. Tune into your own hunger and satiety. Try it on for size and see how it feels. Learning the skills of intuitive eating after years and decades of dieting takes time and patience. You may be tempted to give up and go back to the false safety and temporary comfort of dieting, but remind yourself that the journey is totally worth it.

This can be a difficult and emotional journey, but as the research shows, it can lead to positive rewards in many ways. On page 210 I list my favorite books to help on this journey, but if you feel that you need professional help, seek out a therapist that is trained and aligned with the principles of intuitive eating and Health at Every Size.

Now that you understand the rationale and science behind fostering and teaching intuitive eating to your children, I want to provide you with some guidelines that will help you along the path of intuitive eating for your family.

Chapter 5

The Five Pillars of Healthy Eating

f you want your children to become intuitive eaters, you must set the foundation for success. Here are a few guidelines that provide a framework for feeding your child. I call them the "Five Pillars of Healthy Eating."

1. Honor Hunger and Satiety

Never force a child to eat. Trust them when they say they are no longer hungry and allow them to eat when they are. Forcing a child to eat can be very unpleasant and sometimes even painful to them, especially if they are an intuitive eater. When children are anxious and fearful about a new food, forcing them to eat it leads to feelings of helplessness and distrust and can create the opposite effect you intend—they actually eat *less* and become *more* fearful.

When a child can eat when hungry and stop when full, they will feel more confident to accept a greater variety of foods, won't binge or overeat for fear of scarcity, and will try new foods with less intimidation. Honor your child's unique appetite, eating style, and food preferences. This is a key foundational principle in supporting your child's intuitive eating journey.

I will give you some strategies for approaching "picky eaters" later (see Chapter 17).

Both you and your child have different jobs when it comes to feeding and eating. Think of this as a "division of duties," a concept created by Ellyn Satter in her book, *Child of Mine: Feeding with Love and Good Sense*. Although it changes slightly at each stage of development, the general concept is very simple and easy to remember. As a parent, you have two jobs when it comes to feeding: You decide WHEN and WHAT you will feed your child. Your child also has two jobs: They decide IF and HOW MUCH. This is especially true for younger children. As they grow older, children may take a more significant role in choosing and preparing food, and this will be a beneficial step in their intuitive eating journey. However, you should avoid crossing into their autonomy of how much they choose to eat. It may feel scary at first, but as you get the hang of it, it gets easier and conveys your trust in their eating intuition, allowing them to continue to strengthen these skills over time.

2. Emphasize Whole Plant Foods

In Section 2 of this book I will discuss the benefits of whole plant foods in detail, but the key point is that fruits, vegetables, whole grains, beans, and nuts and seeds in their whole form are packed with vitamins, nutrients, antioxidants, and fiber that promote health and decrease our risk of chronic disease. The more whole plant foods that you include in your family's diet, the better.

3. Establish a Positive Environment

As a parent, it's your role to be the gatekeeper of your household's food culture. This means making the food decisions, planning the menus, and doing the grocery shopping fall under your control. We cannot expect little children to know what is best for their growing bodies and brains. After they enter school and beyond, they'll encounter ample opportunities to have "treats," processed foods, and "party foods" outside the home. For that reason, it is especially important to make the food at home as health-promoting as possible. (Section 2 will explore specific foods that promote health.)

Keep health-promoting foods in the fridge, pantry, and counters, and simply stop filling your refrigerator and cabinets with foods that have little nutritional value. As the gatekeeper, you have a high degree of control over what enters. The exception here is teens who have the independence to purchase and bring home other foods and other adult cohabitants who may not share the same nutritional philosophy—more about that in Chapter 15.

Keep the emphasis on what you place in the house, not what you keep out. In his critically acclaimed book *Mindless Eating*, Brian Wansink recommends keeping health-promoting foods convenient and within view because it really does make a difference in our food choices. Provide an abundance of fruits, vegetables, whole grains, beans, nuts, and seeds on the counter or in other easily accessible and convenient spaces. Place other less healthful foods out of sight where they'll be more difficult to access. In my home, I keep apples, bananas, hummus, whole grain tortillas, unsweetened applesauce, unsweetened peanut butter, and unsalted nuts available for my sons to access when they need a snack after school or before sports.

This does not mean that your home should be devoid of all processed foods, candy, etc. There are ways to approach a healthy balance, and I will go into more detail in the various stages of growth.

Another way to keep the home safe is to avoid dieting and be cautious of the language used in the house concerning body size and shape. In their homes, children should be protected from body shaming, bullying, or teasing and should be sheltered from the influences of media and popular culture that promote the thin ideal.

As we've discussed in previous chapters, dieting is a form of restriction that can create further adverse physical and psychological effects. Never place your child on a diet or hint to them that they should lose weight. Intuitive eating is not a diet, and dieting is not compatible with intuitive eating.

4. Be Flexible

Employ the 80/20 rule. The 80/20 rule means that 80 percent of the time, we strive to eat as healthfully as possible so that we have 20 percent wiggle room to incorporate those foods we usually reserve for celebrations and special occasions. Food can and should be delicious and enjoyable, and pleasure is an essential component of intuitive eating. The world of whole plant foods is enormous, and there are so many delicious recipes and cuisines to explore with our families. However, simple meals are just as delicious. We can teach our children that an apple can be amazing when we are hungry and plain beans and rice can be satisfying and nourishing comfort food. If we act as if health-promoting food is bland and uninteresting, we will pass those beliefs down to our children. Eating can also still be part of special celebrations, holidays, and treats. There is no need to become a purist. It doesn't have to be all-or-nothing! In Chapters 14 to 16, we will discuss how to find balance among these different types of food.

5. Relax and Have Fun!

As parents, we do the best we can. Sometimes we make mistakes, and that's okay. You learn what works and what doesn't as you go. Try not to focus too far into the future and have fun now, especially since each stage of parenting comes with its own set of adventures and challenges. Enjoy exploring new healthy recipes and strategies to integrate healthy habits into your family. And if at first you don't succeed, then try again. Relax, smile, and enjoy the ride! The more relaxed and confident you are about it, the more comfortable and trusting your kids will be. This also means focusing more on the *overall pattern* of your family's habits and well-being instead of focusing on a particular meal or your child's weight or size. Respect your own body and model self-acceptance and self-compassion so that your children learn these skills as well. Don't get hung up on the little details, and please don't try to be perfect. Be joyful and loving to yourself, and you will see how this attitude spreads to the rest of your family.

part II

What to Eat

"Let food be thy medicine and medicine be thy food."

—Hippocrates

Chapter 6

Eating to Thrive

I did not write this book to fearmonger or to cause anxiety over how different foods can lead to health problems. In general, I find it more fruitful and positive to inform others of the beneficial properties of health-promoting foods and how to integrate those foods into their diet. But what I want you to keep in mind is that we live in a world full of risk. There is no way to eradicate risk or exposure to things that create damage over time. Our goal should not be to completely eliminate risk (because that is currently impossible) but to understand how to maximize benefit and minimize risk. At the same time, we want to keep our relationship with food and our bodies healthy and avoid food rules that harm our mental health. Balance, flexibility, adaptability, and moderation are key.

Although intuitive eating does not promote restriction, forcing food, or creating strict food rules, it also does *not* assume that children will naturally know which foods are most health-promoting for them. It is still your job to decide *what* kind of food to offer. There are no perfect diets or "rules" you must follow. However, some foods carry more significant health benefits than others.

For optimal health, center your family's diet around *whole plant* foods. Whole foods are those in their most natural form. Imagine what food would look like if you found it in nature. An example would be an apple picked off a tree. You can discover whole foods in the perimeter of your grocery store, in your garden, and at the farmer's markets. Even if a whole

Surviving vs. Thriving

Humans are natural omnivores. This great advantage has allowed our global population to balloon to almost eight billion people. Humans are so flexible and adaptable that we can survive in diverse and extreme climates and surroundings. Throughout most of human evolution, we have fought to get enough to eat, enduring frequent periods of famine and food scarcity. That is precisely why flexibility in the diet is so advantageous. We have adapted over time to eat just about anything, from tubers, fruits, grains, and legumes to animal flesh, their eggs, and their mammary secretions. Having opposable thumbs, the ability to use tools, and the skills to innovate and learn from our past has given us the unique ability to manipulate our environment (and other animals) to provide food for ourselves. We now grow fruits and vegetables on vast farms and breed millions of animals for food. We've proven that we've mastered our environment, and this has led to greater and more consistent access to food and a higher chance of survival, which in turn, increases the opportunity to live long enough to reproduce and pass our genes down to the next generation. It's incredible and amazing. However, *survival* does not guarantee optimal health or longevity. Surviving does not equal thriving.

More recently, humans have been interested in more than just living long enough to have children. We now want to live and *live well* until old age. We want to feel good during our time on Earth. As parents, we get to choose which foods to bring into our homes to present to our families. Although humans can *survive* on almost any edible substance, I recommend emphasizing those foods that help us *thrive*.

food is placed in a bag or box, it is recognizable and there is usually only one ingredient—the whole food itself! The opposite of whole food is processed food. Processed food is a food that is changed either physically or chemically by grinding it down or adding ingredients such as sugar, salt, fat, or artificial colors, flavors, and preservatives to enhance the color, flavor, and shelf life. Processed food often comes in bags, boxes, or packages and has a long list of ingredients. Fried corn chips and brightly colored children's cereals won't be found in your garden or growing on a tree. The process of refining strips foods of all their health-promoting benefits. In the United States, an estimated 94 percent of our calories come from animal products and processed foods. If you do the math, that only leaves 6 percent for whole plant foods.

What do I mean when I refer to plants? Many people assume that eating plants means just eating salads, fruits, and tasteless "boring" foods. This couldn't be further from the truth! The world of plants is vast and exciting! Whole plant foods include fruits, vegetables, whole grains, beans, nuts, and seeds. The Physicians Committee for Responsible Medicine created the "Power Plate" to represent the foods that should be included in a health-promoting diet. The Power Plate consists of fruits, vegetables, whole grains, and legumes (beans, lentils, and split peas) and represents the foods that we should focus on for good health.

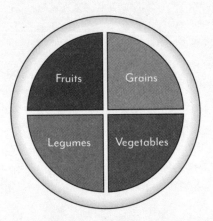

As a Food for Life instructor since 2013, I have been teaching cooking classes and showing adults and children how to incorporate more whole plant foods into their diets in order to prevent and reverse disease. Food for Life is a nutrition education and cooking class program that was created by the Physicians Committee for Responsible Medicine to teach others about the power of diet in chronic disease prevention. I have eaten a plant-based diet since 2011 and was surprised by how much my world of foods has been amplified and expanded. I actually eat a more diverse diet now than I did before I changed my way of eating. Not only has it changed my life, but it has also changed the way I practice pediatrics and how I counsel families about nutrition. Once I discovered the power that whole plant foods have to transform our health and longevity, I became passionate about disseminating this information far and wide.

The Vegan Philosophy

You may have heard the term "vegan." Historically, veganism refers to a philosophy of eating and living that avoids eating or exploiting animals in any way. The term vegan was coined in 1944 by Donald Watson, one of the founders of The Vegan Society. In 1951, the society officially defined veganism as "the doctrine that man should live without exploiting animals." Vegans generally avoid all animal products, including milk, eggs, meats, and honey. They also may choose to avoid purchasing leather and other products made with animal skins or hides. However, those who identify as vegans may not necessarily eat a whole food, plant-based diet.

In contrast, those who choose to eat a whole food, plant-based diet for the health benefits may not identify as vegans. People who eat in this way may refer to themselves as "plant-based" or "whole food plant-based," terms that were created by Dr. T. Colin Campbell in 1982. With the rise in people who choose to eat in this way, the terms have been used interchangeably, but it is helpful to understand the historical origin and differences.

Whole plant foods contain many beneficial components that are vital to our health and are often missing or minimized in animal products and processed foods. Let's review all the ways that whole plant foods can promote health.

Chronic Disease Prevention

When it comes to chronic disease prevention, eating a diet centered on whole plant foods wins the prize. Studies show that eating in this way decreases the risk of cardiovascular disease, diabetes, dementia, cancer, and even mood disorders such as depression and anxiety. In fact, there is evidence that it can potentially reverse heart disease and diabetes and slow the progression of Alzheimer's disease. In his incredibly thorough book, *How Not to Die*, Dr. Michael Greger reviews how whole plant foods are effective in preventing the top fifteen causes of death in the United States. The advantage of whole plant foods is derived not just from what they *lack*, but the nutrients that are bursting from within them.

Macronutrients

In general, all whole plant foods are composed of all three macronutrients: carbohydrates, protein, and fat. In our culture, two of these macronutrients tend to be vilified (carbohydrates and fats), and one of them has been elevated to celebrity status (protein).

I encounter macronutrient fear often. People are either afraid of the dreaded "carbs" or terrified of big, bad fat. However, all macronutrients are needed and utilized in our bodies. There is no need to eliminate or fear any of the macronutrients in whole plant foods. Eating a combination of these nutrients leads to meals that are health-promoting, delicious, and satisfying.

Carbohydrates

In the human body, carbohydrates are broken down into a sugar called glucose. This sugar is the primary source of energy for our muscles and our brain. In fact, glucose is the preferred fuel for our brain because it uses a lot of energy (up to 25 percent of our resting metabolic rate!).

Carbohydrates are found naturally in many foods, including all plant foods. In their whole form, they are called complex carbohydrates. Complex carbohydrates are sugar molecules strung together in long chains. Complex carbohydrates are *only* found in plants. The body must digest and take apart these long chains before they can be absorbed as sugar into the bloodstream.

Complex carbohydrates are often present in "starchy" foods that also contain fiber, and in other nutrients like brown rice, sweet potatoes, squash, and beans. The advantage of complex carbohydrates is that our bodies have to work harder to process them, and they do not get absorbed as quickly into the bloodstream. Complex carbohydrates are more satiating than simple and refined carbohydrates because they come along with other beneficial food components, like fiber and vitamins.

Simple carbohydrates are composed of one or two sugar molecules and are more readily absorbed into the bloodstream. We commonly refer to these as simple sugars. They can be found naturally in fruits, some vegetables, and mammalian milk, including human milk. In contrast, refined sugars are sugars that have been processed and have had fiber and other nutrients stripped from them. Examples include juice and sweeteners such as table sugar, maple syrup, and high fructose corn syrup.

Although they have been vilified, carbohydrates are fundamental to a health-promoting human diet. They give us energy and satisfaction.

Protein

Proteins are chains of molecules called amino acids. Protein is present in all of the cells of the body. Our bodies can make all of the required amino acids, with the exception of nine. These are called essential amino acids because they must be acquired from food.

There is massive anxiety in our society over protein. It comes up in almost every discussion on nutrition. The ironic thing is that most people have never seen or experienced protein deficiency (because it usually only happens in places where people are literally starving to death). Despite this, many also worry that they won't achieve their health or athletic goals if they don't consume sufficient protein.

Although we think of "protein" as animal meat, protein is also abundant in many whole plant foods. Animal flesh doesn't contain only protein but also saturated fat and cholesterol. But even more notable is that animal products are *devoid* of fiber. A whole food, plant-based diet contains sufficient protein, and the protein that is contained in whole plant foods may be more beneficial to humans because it is packaged along with fiber, antioxidants, and water.

Here is my usual response to the concern over protein:

1. Protein is present in *every* whole plant food, in varying percentages. Apples, broccoli, brown rice, and, of course, beans all contain protein. Beans are among the plant foods with the highest protein content, but there is also plenty in leafy greens and vegetables. Forty percent of the calories in broccoli come from protein!

There is a myth floating around that you have to combine certain foods in every meal to absorb adequate protein, but this is false. The human body is intelligent and efficient, and it will take what it needs from various foods, even if they are eaten at different times of the day or week.

2. The average healthy person will absorb enough protein from a variety of whole plant foods as long as they are consuming sufficient calories.

As long as you offer your children a variety of fruits, vegetables, whole grains, and nuts and seeds, and they are eating when they are hungry, they will get enough calories and protein.

Remember, *all* whole plant foods have protein, but because I know you are wondering, here is a list of the categories of plants with the highest protein content in descending order, with examples of high-protein foods in each.

- Legumes: soybeans, tempeh, lentils, black beans, kidney beans, chickpeas

- Nuts: peanut butter, almonds, cashews

- Whole grains: kamut, teff, quinoa, bulgur

- Vegetables: broccoli, spinach, sweet corn, asparagus, brussels sprouts

Not a Food Group

I'd like to take a moment here to vent about a pet peeve I have. Protein is NOT a food group! Protein is one of the basic macronutrients found in a variety of foods. I cringe when I go to a restaurant, and the waiter asks if I would like to add a "protein" to my salad. It is more appropriate to see foods as a source of protein rather than "a protein." Unless you are consuming isolated protein powder, the food you are deriving protein from either contains fiber, vitamins, and antioxidants (whole plants) or saturated fat and cholesterol (animal products) along with the protein contained therein.

Protein is often celebrated in our culture, and it is necessary and important, but it is overemphasized.

Fat

Fat is another macronutrient that our system requires for optimal operation. Fat is found in all of the cells of our body, and it makes up the majority of our brain. In our food, fat comes in many forms: saturated, unsaturated (includes polyunsaturated and monounsaturated), and trans fats. Fatty acids are made up of long carbon chains. Saturation refers to how many hydrogen atoms are bonded to carbon atoms. Saturated fats are generally solid at room temperature while unsaturated fats are liquid. In unsaturated fats, "mono" and "poly" refer to the number of double bonds that are present in the carbon chain. All fats from any origin have varying percentages of saturated and unsaturated fats, but in general, saturated fat is highest in animal products, with the exception of coconut and palm oils. Trans fats are industrially processed fats created by adding hydrogen atoms to vegetable oil to make it solid at room temperature. Examples of trans fats include vegetable shortening and margarine. Trans fats are naturally found in small amounts in meat and dairy, but the majority of trans fats are contained within processed foods such as baked goods, snack foods, and fried foods. Trans fats are harmful to health, and the FDA plans to phase them out of the food supply by January 1, 2021. Although all whole plant foods contain fat, plant foods tend to be naturally low in fat, except for nuts, avocado, coconut, and a few higher fat legumes such as peanuts and soybeans. However, cholesterol is *only* found in animal products and saturated fat is mostly derived from animal foods.

One of the main advantages of fat is its calorie density. Fat is the densest source of calories, giving us nine calories per gram. Both carbohydrates and proteins have only four calories per gram. Fats also provide us with essential fatty acids and optimize our absorption of fat-soluble vitamins (A, D, E, K). Fat is the most efficient form of storage in our body, allowing us to store thousands of calories to use in times of need.

Fat is very satisfying and delicious as it contributes flavor and mouthfeel to a pleasurable meal. However, when derived from whole plant foods it also contains fiber, antioxidants, and other nutrients for bonus benefits.

Micronutrients: Vitamins and Minerals

Micronutrients are essential vitamins, minerals, and phytochemicals that our bodies need and use to perform many necessary functions. Examples of micronutrients include vitamins A, C, D, E, K, multiple B vitamins, iron, zinc, and calcium, all of which are vital to the proper functioning of our bodies. They are called micronutrients because we need only consume them in small amounts (usually in the order of milligrams, as opposed to macronutrients, which we require many grams of per day), yet not having enough can lead to deficiency and health problems. We obtain the majority of our vitamins and minerals from food and water.

Those on vegetarian or vegan diets tend to consume larger quantities of vitamin A, vitamin C, vitamin E, folate, magnesium, and niacin. In a randomized controlled clinical trial of people with type 2 diabetes, participants who consumed a vegan diet had improved dietary quality overall with increased intake of vitamin A, beta-carotene, vitamin C, vitamin K, folate, magnesium, and potassium.

Maximize Nutrient Intake

Dr. Joel Fuhrman is a physician and author of the best seller *Eat to Live*. He coined the term "nutritarian" to describe a way of eating that focuses on eating foods that are high in nutrient density. Nutrient density refers to the concentration of micronutrients (vitamins, minerals, and phytochemicals) per calorie. Dr. Fuhrman recommends that humans eat G-BOMBS daily (greens, berries, onions, mushrooms, beans, and seeds) to maximize nutrient intake.

Antioxidants

Another beneficial substance we can obtain from food are antioxidants. Antioxidants help prevent oxidation, a chemical reaction that causes damage to cells. This cellular damage, over time, can lead to mutations that are the precursors to cancer, chronic diseases such as diabetes and heart disease, as well as signs of aging.

There are many different antioxidants, but some of the more well-known include beta-carotene, vitamin A, vitamin C, and vitamin E. However, hundreds of different nutrients act as antioxidants, and they are derived from various plant foods. The more colorful, the better. This is why eating "from the rainbow" is so beneficial.

Get Your Antioxidants from
FOOD, Not Supplements!

One word of caution. After hearing all the great benefits of antioxidants, you may be tempted to run out and buy your kids some antioxidant gummy vitamins (seriously, it seems like everything is in gummy form these days). Not so fast! Studies have shown that most antioxidant supplements are not beneficial, and they may actually be harmful. Whenever we obtain our antioxidants from *food*, we are eating them along with many other beneficial vitamins and nutrients that likely work together to produce the health benefits that occur in our bodies.

Plants have some pretty impressive properties. They are *packed* with antioxidants, phytochemicals, and vitamins. Carotenoids are a group of antioxidants found in yellow, orange, and red fruits and vegetables. They promote healthy vision, support the immune system, and have a role in cancer prevention. Lycopene is a carotenoid found in tomatoes and has been found to decrease the risk of prostate cancer. One fascinating study found that those who eat a diet higher in fruits and vegetables have detectable levels of carotenoids in their skin. You really are what you eat!

Many people are surprised that herbs and spices have the biggest "bang for your buck" when it comes to antioxidants. However, antioxidants are found in all whole plant foods, so you can't go wrong. Below is a list of food categories with the greatest antioxidant potential, in descending order, and some examples of foods in each of those categories.

- Spices: cloves, oregano, ginger, turmeric, cinnamon, curry
- Herbs: basil, parsley, cilantro, rosemary, thyme
- Berries: blueberries, raspberries, blackberries, cranberries, strawberries
- Leafy greens: kale, spinach, collard greens, rainbow chard, bok choy
- Beans: black beans, red beans, kidney beans, pinto beans
- Vegetables: artichokes, eggplants, sweet potatoes
- Fruit: apples, cherries, plums

One way to determine the antioxidant potential of a food is through its ORAC score. ORAC stands for "oxygen radical absorbance capacity," and it was created by researchers at the National Institutes of Health and the National Institute on Aging to determine the antioxidant content of certain foods. Animal products contain minimal antioxidants, and the antioxidants they do provide come from the plants that the animals themselves eat. On average, plant foods contain sixty-four times more antioxidants than anything derived from an animal.

Fiber

Fiber is my favorite "f" word. I talk about it as much as possible. Hopefully, after you learn about its superpowers, you will too! In the standard American diet, fiber is often neglected and is likely one of our most significant deficiencies. Modern diets are low in fiber because of food processing, which often strips whole plant foods of their fiber. Fiber deficiency creates some obvious health problems such as constipation, but it is likely also leaving us more vulnerable to chronic disease.

Fiber is plant roughage and is technically a carbohydrate. However, because the human body cannot digest it, it passes through our system unabsorbed. In other words, it does not contribute to calorie intake. It may seem inert, but fiber has some amazing properties.

There are two types of fiber—soluble and insoluble—and they each have distinctive properties. Soluble fiber is the type that dissolves in water. Insoluble fiber does not dissolve and contributes to the bulk in our bowel movements.

It is recommended that adults consume around 30 grams of fiber per day. The recommended intake for children increases with age, starting with about 19 grams per day for toddlers and increasing to adult levels by adolescence. However, most adults in the US consume only 15 grams of fiber or less per day on average, and only 5 percent of the US population meets the current recommendations for fiber intake.

Why am I so obsessed with fiber? There are at least four vital functions of fiber that promote health and fight disease.

1. Fiber helps keep our digestive system regular. Because fiber is plant roughage, it helps attract and bind water, which leads to soft, easy-to-pass stools. Constipation is a common chronic condition in both children and adults that could be relieved by increasing fiber in the diet.

2. Fiber helps remove toxins, excess hormones, and cholesterol. Soluble fiber can decrease our risk of chronic disease through a fascinating mechanism. It binds to cholesterol and excess hormones that circulate through our bodies. Once these particles are attached to the fiber, they are removed with our waste.

3. Fiber contributes to satiety. Insoluble fiber contributes to fullness both during a meal and afterward. In other words, meals that contain more fiber are going to help us feel more satisfied because fiber helps create volume and bulk. It also blunts the rise of blood sugar levels after we eat a meal.

4. Fiber promotes the growth and maintenance of healthy gut bacteria. Plant foods are both prebiotic and probiotic. Probiotics are foods or substances that contain live microorganisms that are thought to be beneficial to the human body. Alternatively, prebiotics are foods or substances that feed these healthy microorganisms in order to promote their growth and survival. Whole plant foods are prebiotic when they provide fiber for beneficial gut bacteria to consume and, when fermented or cultured, plants are probiotic and can directly replenish our gut bacteria. Examples of common probiotic plant foods are yogurt, tempeh, kimchi, miso, and sauerkraut. We are now recognizing the importance of the symbiotic bacteria that live in our digestive system and contribute to our gut health. Probiotics are being increasingly used to treat infant colic, antibiotic-associated diarrhea, and viral gastroenteritis.

a parent's guide to intuitive eating

Where Gas Comes From

Speaking of bacteria...do you know where gas comes from? Many people are embarrassed about gas and, because of that, they may avoid high-fiber foods such as beans. However, our beneficial gut bacteria digest the fiber in these foods and produce these gasses, so we should be happy when we have more toots! It means that we are feeding our symbiotic friends, and, in turn, they will help us.

When we eat whole plant foods, we promote the growth of beneficial gut bacteria. However, harmful gut bacteria can also colonize our gut. Recent studies have shown that our gut bacteria produce byproducts that can either help us or hurt us. In fact, harmful gut bacteria may even contribute to heart disease and mental illness! One harmful byproduct is called trimethylamine N-oxide, also known as TMAO, and is formed when gut bacteria digest red meat. This byproduct can increase the risk of heart disease and strokes. Research scientists have found significant differences in the types of bacteria in the guts of people with depression versus those who were not depressed. Gut bacteria can produce and release neuroactive chemicals such as serotonin, which is a neurotransmitter that is typically low in depression. We are still learning how these little bugs interact with our bodies, but we do know that we can increase our good gut bacteria and decrease our bad ones by eating more whole plant foods! So, remember, if you have gas, smile knowing that you are feeding your friendly bacteria.

I can't help but think of that song and how true it is: "Beans, beans, the magical food, the more you eat, the more you toot. The more you toot, the better you feel, so eat beans with every meal!"

We must eat plant foods in their whole form to obtain sufficient fiber. It is well known that those who consume a plant-based diet have a higher intake of fiber. Most whole plants have varying degrees of both types of fiber. However, the best bang for your buck when loading up on fiber comes in the form of beans. In descending order, below are the categories of plant foods with the highest fiber per serving:

- Legumes (beans, split peas, and lentils): 7 grams per ½ cup

- Leafy greens: 4 grams per cup

- Vegetables: 4 grams per cup

- Whole grains: 3 to 4 grams per cup

- Fruits: 3 grams per cup

Fiber should come from your food, not a bottle. Avoid the fiber gummies and the Metamucil and eat more whole plants instead! The superpower of plant foods is fiber. Fiber is ONLY found in plants, including ALL whole plant foods.

Water

The human body requires water for survival, proper function, health, and well-being. In fact, 60 percent of the human body is composed of water. We derive our water from the beverages that we drink and the food that we eat. The Institute of Medicine estimates that about 20 percent of our total daily water intake is derived from food.

In addition to being used by every cell in the body, water helps regulate temperature, maintain blood pressure, and flush out wastes and toxins through urine. It also contributes to healthy digestion, lubricates joints, and keeps mucous membranes and skin hydrated. Even mild dehydration can affect mood and lead to irritability and low energy. This happens because the brain needs water to function optimally—it is composed of 73 percent water! Moreover, dehydration affects the transport of electrolytes, which can lead to muscle weakness or cramping. Hydrating adequately gives us energy, helps us think better, and even affects the appearance of our skin. Consuming adequate water also ensures that fiber can do its work properly.

Another highly beneficial property of water in our food is satiety, especially when it is combined with fiber (my favorite!). And water has no calories! Foods that are naturally high in water content are usually low in calories. All whole plant foods contain water. In fact, most fresh fruits and vegetables are composed of at least 80 percent water. Active children may also benefit from eating high water fruits to maintain proper hydration, especially when they don't want to slow down to drink water.

As you can see, food does much more than just give us fuel. When we consume foods that are composed of carbohydrates, protein, fat, are rich in vitamins, minerals, antioxidants, fiber, and contain water, we can nourish all the cells and systems of our bodies for optimal functioning and also decrease the risk of disease.

Is It Safe?

For many years vegetarian and vegan diets were seen as lacking in nutrition. Even to this day, many health-care providers may not know of current research that debunks this myth and validates the health-promoting potential of a plant-centric diet. The Academy of Nutrition and Dietetics, which is made up of food and nutrition professionals such as registered dietitians, states: "Appropriately planned vegetarian, including vegan, diets are healthful, nutritionally adequate, and may provide health benefits in the prevention and treatment of certain diseases. These diets are appropriate for all stages of the life cycle, including pregnancy, lactation, infancy, childhood, adolescence, older adulthood, and for athletes. Plant-based diets are more environmentally sustainable than diets rich in animal products because they use fewer natural resources and are associated with much less environmental damage."

Caring for Our Planet:
Our Diet Doesn't Affect Just Us

Although it may not be directly related to our health, being conscious of the effect that our food choices have on the planet and on other creatures will benefit our world. Currently, many global organizations are urging people to eat less meat and more plants. The reason is simple. Raising animals for our consumption is straining our planet and draining our natural resources. As we approach a global population of eight billion people and our appetite for animal products increases, Mother Earth is struggling to keep up. The meat and dairy industries currently use a third of the Earth's fresh water, and livestock cover 45 percent of the world's total land. Animal agriculture also produces tremendous waste, some of which is toxic to the earth, the sea, and humans.

A person who eats a plant-based diet produces 50 percent less carbon dioxide and uses 1/13th of the water and 1/18th of the land a meat eater does. Even if you don't choose to eat plants 100 percent of the time, the more plants you eat and the less animal products you consume, the more you are supporting a healthy ecosystem that will sustain us for centuries to come. Teach your children about this too! You may be surprised how interested they are in caring for their home planet and how they may encourage you to make more choices that are aligned with this goal.

Teaching Compassion

By the time we are adults, we tend to become desensitized to many of the customs and practices around us because "it's just the way it's done." Because of this, we tend to teach these same practices to our children and grandchildren. When we stop to look at the world through a child's eyes, we may see things in a different light. We have eaten animals since the beginning of humanity. There are likely times in our evolution that we would have perished had we not been omnivorous. However, in this country, we no longer face frequent famines, and our booming population and pressing demand for animal products has led to a business of meat, dairy, and egg production that is massive and, often, cruel. Every day in our world, 150 million land animals are killed for food. This doesn't include the over two billion farmed and wild-caught fish that are killed daily. Most children are naturally compassionate toward animals and desire not to hurt them. If we take a child's perspective, maybe we can also see that the suffering that we are causing is not all necessary. We can teach them about the food industry and how we can make choices that will ultimately lead to less suffering for the animals that are bred for food. Purchasing more humanely raised and slaughtered animals is a choice, but an even better option is to simply put less demand on the system and eat less meat, dairy, and eggs. This simple choice to eat *less* benefits the planet, shows compassion for the animals, and increases our health and well-being.

Other countries are starting to recognize the rise of plant-based diets and have created literature to guide and reassure health-care providers. In 2019, Italian authors released "Vegan Nutrition for Mothers and Children," which states, "The growth of vegan preschoolers, children, and adolescents falls within normal range.... Children following plant-based diets might have lower risk of developing obesity, are less exposed to veterinary antibiotics found in animal-derived foods, and show a more favorable anti-inflammatory adipokine profile." Adipokines are cell-signaling proteins that are secreted by fat tissue and communicate with the rest of the body. In a 2010 paper discussing different types of vegetarian diets in children and adolescents, the Canadian Paediatric Society states, "A well-balanced vegetarian diet as a healthy lifestyle choice is an acceptable option to provide for the needs of growth and development in the young." A long-term study published in 1988 on the growth and development of vegan British children found that "provided sufficient care is taken, a vegan diet can support normal growth and development."

A plant-based diet is nutritious and safe for children and adults. I have raised my own children on a plant-based diet and have no concerns about recommending it to my patients.

Integrating a Plant-Centered Diet

If you have read this far and are starting to have major anxiety, thinking, "I could never go 100 percent plant-based!" please pause and take a deep breath. No evidence shows you have to be 100 percent plant-based to lead a healthy lifestyle and decrease the risk of disease. However, we know that eating a diet composed *mostly* of animal products and processed foods DOES increase your risk of disease. So perhaps the answer is somewhere in the middle?

Studies of the Blue Zones (places in the world where people are naturally living long, healthy lives into their nineties and one hundreds) demonstrate a correlation between eating a predominantly plant-based diet and longevity. People in the Blue Zones generally eat meat just a few times per month and include legumes (beans, lentils, split peas) in their diet.

I realize that eating a purely plant-based diet is not feasible nor desirable for everyone. For those who do not choose to eat entirely plant-based, I recommend aiming for a target of 75 percent. This would mean that you eat animal products in up to five meals per week, but the goal for the rest of the meals would be to load up on fruits, vegetables, whole grains, beans, and nuts and seeds. If you aren't sure where to start, below are several approaches that help you integrate more whole plant foods into your diet.

- **Meatless Monday (or Tuesday, Wednesday, Thursday...)**. Begin by eating fully plant-based one day per week and work up from there. On other days of the week, find little ways to add more fruits, vegetables, whole grains, beans, and nuts and seeds to all of your meals. Once you get comfortable with that, you can add more days to your plan.

- **The "Weekday Vegan."** In this approach, all of your meals Monday through Friday are plant-based so that your weekend can be more flexible. For some families this may be easier and more flexible to accommodate for dining out and social events that occur on weekends.

- **The "Vegan before 6."** Alternatively, you can choose to make all of your breakfasts and lunches plant-based so you can be more relaxed at dinner.

What do plant-based meals look like? It's actually simpler than you might think and you probably consume many of these foods already! Here are a few ideas for meals and snacks:

Breakfast

- Oatmeal cooked in water or plant-based milk (such as almond, coconut, hemp, or soy milk) topped with blueberries and walnuts
- Fruity Roll-Ups: whole wheat tortilla with natural peanut butter (or other nut or seed butter) stuffed with sliced bananas and strawberries (see page 165)
- Whole grain cold cereal with soy milk and fruit
- Avocado toast with sliced tomatoes
- Green smoothie with a bran muffin

Lunch

- Peanut butter and jelly sandwich with an apple or banana (a classic!)
- Bagel sandwich smothered with roasted red pepper hummus and layered with sliced cucumbers, tomatoes, and onion
- Bean burrito filled with refried pinto beans, salsa, and guacamole
- Veggie corn tacos stuffed with black beans, corn, and fresh avocado
- Dairy-free tomato soup with crusty bread

Dinner

- Whole grain pasta with marinara sauce and roasted vegetables

- Cuban black beans, rice, and a side salad

- Veggie burger on a whole wheat bun with all the trimmings and baked sweet potato fries

- Loaded veggie pizza made with whole grain crust, red sauce, chickpeas, and all your favorite veggies

- Veggie sushi and miso soup

Snacks

- Fresh fruit (apples, pears, bananas, plums, oranges...the choices are endless!)

- Raw, cut-up veggies (carrots, broccoli, cauliflower, red bell peppers) dipped in hummus

- Crispy roasted chickpeas

- Homemade trail mix (raw unsalted nuts with dried fruit)

- Leftovers from breakfast, lunch, or dinner

No matter where you are, just remember to do the best that you can to incorporate more whole plant foods (fruits, vegetables, whole grains, beans, and nuts and seeds) into every meal and every day. There is no right or wrong approach. Do what you can and tweak your approach over time. See it as a fun challenge. After a while, it will become second nature. Remember that you are the boss and the ultimate gatekeeper of the nutrition of your household.

If your child doesn't like vegetables and it feels like a momentous task to encourage them to eat them, don't worry, you won't be forcing broccoli on your kid. I will give you strategies for introducing more vegetables and fruits to your children in the next section, but before then, I think it is valuable to understand how tastes develop.

How Tastes Develop

Babies are born with a preference for breast milk. Besides that, every other taste preference is acquired. The process of developing a taste for a specific food demands exposure—*repeated, persistent, exposure.* We build our inclinations for food by experiencing it over and over again. Some taste preferences may even seem extreme, and yet, they develop. As I said before, humans are remarkably adaptable and have learned to survive in a wide variety of places on Earth. From these different geographical locations, a diversity of flavors and textures of foods have blossomed. Children in Mexico grow up eating beans and rice and tortillas with hot sauce. Children in India are raised on robust curries and very spicy foods. In other countries, most children start to eat what their parents eat as soon as they start solids. They don't get a different menu. However, in the United States, we have assumed that children eat a very special diet that consists of chicken nuggets, French fries, grilled cheese sandwiches, and the strict exclusion of anything green or sharp in flavor. Because a child may reject vegetables once or twice (or many more times), parents assume that it is a food that children will not like and stop offering it. In *First Bite*, author Bee Wilson writes how personal food habits are shaped: "Our responses to food are remarkably open to influence and remain so throughout our lives." She goes on to write, "To a large extent, children eat—and therefore like—what's in front of them, particularly in conditions of scarcity."

No matter how old you are, you *can* learn to like and even love new foods. Believe it or not, your brain and your taste buds can adapt to changes in your diet through a process called neuroadaptation. Neuroadaptation is especially apparent to individuals when they transition from a diet that is high in processed foods packed with sugar, salt, and fat to a more natural diet based on whole foods. At first, the whole, natural foods may seem tasteless and not stimulating enough, but after time, sometimes in as little as a few days, the brain adapts to the change, and the new foods begin to taste better. This works exceptionally well when one uses hunger to their advantage and eats when the body is ready to accept and digest food.

The human body is built to eat a variety of whole plant foods. Even if your child avoids certain foods often, as you start to integrate more health-promoting foods into the diet and repeatedly expose them to these foods, they WILL develop a taste for them and may even come to love them. I promise!

Chapter 7

Nutrients of Concern

M any people worry that eating a certain way will lead to deficiencies that can lead to health problems. That is a valid concern. Like I said before, there is no perfect diet, and certain nutrients should be supplemented no matter what style of eating you adopt. In this chapter, I'll discuss what's often left out of the conversation: the most common deficiencies in the standard American diet and how a diet centered around whole plant foods will actually create vitamin and nutrient *advantages* that improve your health, well-being, and longevity.

Iron

Iron is a nutrient of concern for the entire population of the planet. Iron is a heavy metal that is necessary for the formation of hemoglobin, an essential component of red blood cells. Because of this, iron deficiency can lead to a medical condition called anemia. Anemia is when you have fewer blood cells than you need to transport oxygen in your bloodstream adequately. It can lead to fatigue, pale skin, rapid heart rate, and not feeling well in general. Anemia affects nearly a third of the world's population, with women and children in resource-poor countries being the greatest affected. Globally, at least half of all anemia is caused by iron deficiency.

Although iron deficiency is the most common nutrient deficiency in the United States, it is a myth that vegan and vegetarian children suffer more from iron-deficiency anemia than omnivorous children. You do not need to eat meat to obtain sufficient iron. Although vegetarians and vegans may have lower iron stores overall, they do not tend to have increased rates of anemia. Iron is plentiful in beans and leafy greens. The iron found in plants is called non-heme iron. In contrast, heme iron is derived from animal meat. "Heme" indicates that the iron is already bound to a heme protein. Iron absorption is aided by the simultaneous ingestion of vitamin C, which is also plentiful in fruits and vegetables.

Other causes of iron deficiency are iron loss or decreased absorption of iron, which can occur when consuming excess dairy. Cow's milk can cause microscopic bleeding in the guts of infants. This slow, asymptomatic bleeding over time can lead to the loss of iron. This is why it is advised to not introduce cow's milk to children under one year of age. Dairy is also naturally low in iron, so when children consume excess milk and dairy, they are displacing foods that are naturally rich in iron. Additionally, dairy protein tends to block the absorption of iron from other sources.

Teen girls and women are at greater risk of iron-deficiency anemia because they experience monthly blood loss through menstruation. Typically, this occurs in women who have heavy or prolonged periods that lead to excessive blood loss (thus, the loss of iron), and the body can't keep up with manufacturing enough new blood cells without enough raw materials.

It is also not commonly known that coffee and black tea have properties that block the absorption of iron when consumed with meals. Hopefully your kiddos aren't consuming caffeine, but in the South, sweet tea is pretty standard, and some teens do start drinking coffee regularly.

Despite all of the different ways one can become iron deficient, obtaining sufficient iron on a plant-based diet is not difficult or complicated. The best sources of iron in a plant-based diet include legumes, leafy greens, and some whole grains. Below is a list of plant foods with high iron content in each plant category.

- Beans and lentils: lentils, soybeans, tofu, tempeh, lima beans

- Nuts and seeds: pumpkin seeds, pine nuts, pistachios, sunflower seeds, cashews, unhulled sesame seeds, hemp seeds, flaxseeds

- Vegetables: tomato sauce, spinach, kale, swiss chard, collard greens

- Cereals and grains: quinoa, fortified cereals, brown rice, oatmeal

- Other: blackstrap molasses, prune juice, dark chocolate

Calcium

Calcium is a vitamin that, along with vitamin D, is necessary for the proper development of bones, a process that is tightly regulated in the body. It is also required for the electrical conduction within heart cells and the proper function of neurotransmitters. When you hear the word calcium, what is the first food you think of? Most people automatically think of milk. I grew up in the age of "Milk, it does the body good" commercials. I LOVED the stuff and often drank a glass with each meal, with snacks, and in my many, many bowls of sugary cereal. Yes, milk does contain calcium. However, it is not the only source of calcium in the human diet, and it is certainly not essential for the development of strong, healthy bones.

A Word about Dairy and Why I Don't Love It

I take a very gentle approach when discussing nutrition with my families. I emphasize the benefits of whole plant foods but do not condemn patients or families for eating animal products. However, I struggle with dairy. The irony of the entire situation is that dairy used to be one of my favorite food groups. I loved butter, cream, and ice cream—the thicker and creamier, the better. My family owns a large dairy farm. I grew up hearing and believing that dairy was a miracle food and essential for proper growth and development. And as a young pediatrician, I preached the necessity of a minimum of two to three servings of dairy every day, especially for girls. I now look back and realize how I had just been repeating a cultural dogma. I saw how milk was harming children, from severe anemia and chronic constipation to abdominal pain, lactose intolerance, and babies that had bloody stools from cow's milk protein intolerance.

Then I began to understand the connection between dairy, acne, and menstrual pain. Many patients have shown improvements in their autoimmune conditions, arthritis, and other symptoms when they stopped consuming dairy. Because cow's milk is made for baby cows, the human body can react negatively to the protein, which can lead to adverse effects. Once I learned more about it and saw the evidence, I began to see dairy in a completely different light. I get it. Dairy really does taste delicious. But I can no longer claim that it is a health food. Dairy is not necessary for children and adults, and it can cause harm. I now counsel families to limit the intake of dairy in their children, but if you are able to remove it from the diet completely, do it, especially if your child is experiencing any adverse effects from it. If not, then see it as a "play" food that does not have a central part in your diet. Definitely allow no more than two total servings per day. One serving of dairy is 8 ounces of milk, 4 ounces of yogurt, 1 ounce of cheese, or ½ cup of ice cream. However, these days there are so many great dairy alternatives available, even in small towns such as ours, that avoiding dairy is really not as hard as it used to be. But some children should avoid it completely for health reasons, including those with chronic abdominal pain and chronic constipation.

Here are two thoughts on calcium and healthy bone development:

1. Calcium is present and absorbable in many whole plant foods! It is especially high in beans and greens.

Plant foods high in absorbable calcium:

- Leafy greens: collard greens, turnip greens, kale, bok choy, broccoli, cabbage

- Beans: tofu, tempeh, soybeans, navy beans, chickpeas

- Other: tahini, almond butter, blackstrap molasses

- Fortified foods: fortified plant-based milks

2. The best way to build strong bones and prevent bone loss is through weight-bearing exercise and *adequate* calcium intake. No matter how much milk or calcium you consume, if you don't stress the bones through exercise, you will not build your bones to their highest potential. Children are naturally active and want to play and run. Let them be children! Let them use the monkey bars and climb because this is the way they build strong bones and muscles.

Lactose Intolerance

Lactose is present in mammalian milk, but we encounter it most frequently in cow's milk. Lactose intolerance is rare in babies, but relatively common among adults. It is more common in certain ethnic groups than others. Around 65 percent of humans have decreased lactase activity after infancy, but in some East Asian communities lactose intolerance can be as high as 90 percent.

Lactase is an enzyme that breaks down lactose and allows us to digest it. We are born with sufficient lactase because human milk also contains lactose. However, the production of lactase starts to decrease around the time of weaning. When we are unable to break down and digest lactose, it causes gastrointestinal bloating, pain, diarrhea, or constipation and flatulence.

Supplements

Contrary to popular belief, most vitamins and supplements do not improve health or make up for major errors in our diet. Although supplements can prevent deficiencies in micronutrients, they are meant to complement a diet with a strong foundation. However, a few are worth deliberately including in your regimen.

Vitamin B12

Vitamin B12 is necessary for the development of healthy blood cells. It is also utilized in the nervous system in the formation of myelin, the sheaths of insulation around nerves. This vitamin is an essential supplement for everyone who consumes an exclusively plant-based diet. Vitamin B12 is only produced by certain bacteria present in the soil. In the past, we likely consumed more B12 because we ate unwashed food that naturally contained more of these bacteria. However, ruminant animals such as cows that eat grass ingest these bacteria. The bacteria become part of their gut flora and continue to produce vitamin B12, which is then stored in their muscles and organs. That is why meat eaters are less likely to develop vitamin B12 deficiency. However, as we age, we are less able to absorb B12 even from meat, so the Institute of Medicine recommends that all adults over the age of fifty take vitamin B12. You can take vitamin B12 by itself in sublingual or liquid form, or take it as part of a daily multivitamin. For children, I recommend 500mg per day or 1000mcg two to three times per week. Alternatively, you can give them a daily multivitamin that contains B12.

Foods commonly fortified with B12 include plant-based milks and nutritional yeast. I recommend that babies born to vegan mothers start taking the supplement after birth and that vegan mothers continue to supplement themselves during breastfeeding.

Vitamin D

Vitamin D is a hormone that is produced in the skin with exposure to sunlight. It is essential for the development of strong bones. People who live in sunny regions may not have difficulty producing sufficient vitamin D as long as they are exposed to sunlight for twenty to thirty minutes per day. However, in many parts of the United States and during certain times of the year, it may be challenging to obtain sufficient sunlight. We spend much more time indoors now than we used to, and we also use more clothing and often wear sunblock. In my home state of Washington, the days are short during the fall and winter months. To obtain sufficient sun exposure for adequate vitamin D production, a person would have to stand outside with arms and legs exposed for two hours in the middle of the day. In the United States, those who live north of the 37th parallel are at greater risk for deficiency in the fall and winter. Those with a darker complexion may require even more time in the sun to produce sufficient vitamin D. This is why it is advisable for most children to consume a daily vitamin D supplement of at least 400 to 600 IU per day. It is recommended that babies be supplemented with vitamin D after birth to prevent a softening of the bones, called rickets. Alternatively, a breastfeeding mother can take a daily dose of 6,400 IU of vitamin D to ensure that the baby acquires sufficient vitamin D.

Many people have been told that cow's milk is a good source of vitamin D. Cow's milk is naturally low in vitamin D and becomes even lower through processing. This is why it has to be "fortified" with vitamin D. Supplementing through a vitamin is a more reliable way of ensuring that you and your child are consuming sufficient vitamin D and allows you to skip the milk.

One whole plant food contains vitamin D: mushrooms! Mushrooms exposed to UV light produce vitamin D similarly to how humans produce it from sunlight. A 3-ounce serving of mushrooms that have been UV treated could contain 400 IU of vitamin D2! Vitamin D2 is known as ergocalciferol and is derived from plants. Cholecalciferol is also known as Vitamin D3, and it is derived from animal products. Most supplements are made from the D2 form.

Although the data on vitamin D deficiency is mixed, evidence shows that vitamin D deficiency is rampant. Supplementing vitamin D does not seem to cause harm or toxicity, so it seems prudent and cautious to supplement this vitamin to prevent potential deficiency.

Omega-3 Fatty Acids

Omega-3 fatty acids are required for proper brain development and a healthy cardiovascular system. Omega-3 fatty acids come in the form of alpha-linolenic acid (ALA), eicosapentaenoic acid (EPA), and docosahexaenoic acid (DHA).

Omega-3 fatty acids naturally occur in some whole plants, particularly flaxseeds, raw walnuts, chia seeds, and hemp seeds. They are also present in leafy greens such as kale. Incorporating these foods into the diet is a good idea and doesn't have to be complicated. To absorb significant omega-3 fatty acids from flaxseeds, they must be ground. It is also important to keep ground flaxseeds cool and away from direct light exposure as the fats can go rancid. I keep mine in my freezer. Adding a ground tablespoon to oatmeal, smoothies, or baked goods is an easy and yummy way to incorporate flax. The type of omega-3 fatty acids found in these plants is the ALA type. Many people can convert a small percentage of ALA into DHA and EPA, but some can't. Because of that, it might be beneficial to supplement DHA and EPA. At this time, there are no official guidelines for recommended dietary allowance for omega-3 fatty acids, but this is an area of evolving research.

For many years it was advised to take fish oil for heart disease prevention. However, fish oil may not be beneficial for at least one reason. Because fish oil is derived from fish fat, it can be contaminated with mercury. For this reason, make sure to choose either a vegan omega-3 supplement or fish oil that has been tested and does not contain mercury.

The good news is that DHA and EPA omega-3 fatty acids are produced by microalgae. Algal oil can be derived from these microalgae and consumed as a supplement. Interestingly, the omega-3 fatty acids found in fish fat actually come from these algae. The fish end up with the omega-3 fat because they eat the algae (or they eat the fish that eat the algae).

Good plant-based sources of omega-3 fatty acids:

- Ground flaxseeds
- Hemp seeds
- Chia seeds
- Walnuts
- Leafy greens (kale, spinach, broccoli, brussels sprouts)
- Algal oil supplement in liquid or capsule form

Multivitamins

Many multivitamins usually do contain the nutrients of concern in adequate amounts. The only things that are not routinely added to a multivitamin are the DHA/EPA omega-3 fatty acids. Parents ask me all the time for brand recommendations, and I have to admit there are so many supplement brands that I don't have time to look into all of them. In general, I look for brands that do not have any added animal products, especially dairy. There are several brands that I trust and have used for myself and my family, including Dr. Fuhrman's line of vitamins, Complement, and Complement Plus by Alpine Organics. The spray called "Complement" contains just B12, vitamin D, and omega-3 DHA/EPA. They also have a capsule that is called "Complement Plus," which has everything I discussed above, including the omega-3. However, this will not work well for small children as it has to be swallowed whole. Another omega-3 DHA/EPA in liquid I have used is Omega Zen.

part III

Setting the Table for Healthy Eating Habits

Good habits are worth being fanatical about.

—John Irving, American novelist

Chapter 8

Lifestyle Habits That Support Intuitive Eating

You've learned what intuitive eating is and why it helps keep children healthy and happy. You've also learned about food and how it can benefit us, and what foods maximize benefits and decrease the risk of chronic disease. Before I delve into specific techniques that you can apply to feeding your child, I want to cover three lifestyle habits that will ultimately support your intuitive eating journey.

As I have previously explained, our eating behaviors are very complex and driven by a multitude of factors. Choosing health-promoting foods and using the principles of intuitive eating to guide you will undoubtedly be beneficial. However, other lifestyle habits also affect our bodies, our appetites, and our metabolism. You can optimize these distinct areas in your family to contribute to the overall goal of raising healthy and happy children.

Sleep

I believe that sleep is becoming one of the most abused lifestyle habits in the modern era. Artificial lighting, television, video games, and social media all contribute to keeping us awake longer than we naturally would and can lead to chronic, habitual sleep deprivation. The amount of sleep deprivation that children experience really worries me, and because of this, I spend a lot of time counseling families on the importance of adequate sleep.

Why Do We Need Sleep?

We spend about a third of our lives sleeping. But sleep isn't wasted time. It is incredibly valuable and necessary for our brains and bodies to function properly. We need rest to process memories, form secure neural connections, and remove toxins from our brains that build up during waking hours. Children require a lot of sleep throughout their lives, and it is critical for proper growth and development. It is essential that children acquire sufficient sleep each night and that they have a regular, consistent bedtime routine.

How Sleep Deprivation Affects Our Metabolism and Eating Behaviors

Chronic sleep deprivation affects our metabolism in more than one way. It decreases our resting energy expenditure so that we burn fewer calories at rest, makes us more resistant to insulin, raises our insulin levels, and increases our appetite so that we actually *want* to eat more. Spending more hours awake increases the time for eating opportunities. Sleep deprivation directly affects our appetite hormones, increasing hunger hormones and decreasing satiety hormones. This is an unfortunate combination of effects and, over time, can lead to weight gain and excess body fat. But the critical point here is that if your child is sleep-deprived, they are going to be compelled to eat, usually foods that are high in sugar, fat, and salt.

Other Consequences of Sleep Deprivation

Of course, sleep deprivation can also cause a plethora of other undesirable effects such as irritability, depression, anxiety, difficulty concentrating, and behavior problems. Sleep deprivation increases our risk of developing Alzheimer's disease decades later. Sleep is essential. Please don't neglect it, and take care to foster excellent sleep habits in your children.

Sleep Requirements in Children (per 24 hours)*

4 to 12 months	12 to 16 hours (includes naps)
1 to 2 years	11 to 14 hours (includes naps)
3 to 5 years	10 to 13 hours (includes naps)
6 to 12 years	9 to 12 hours
13 to 18 years	8 to 10 hours

*From American Academy of Sleep Medicine and American Academy of Pediatrics

How Do You Know If Your Child Is Getting Enough Sleep?

Although there are general guidelines about how much sleep a person needs at different ages, everyone is different and may fall at various places in the spectrum of sleep requirements.

If your child appears refreshed and energetic after they wake in the morning, it is a sign that they have had enough restorative sleep. There are definitely different personality types, and not all children are going to be "morning people." But if your child has a hard time waking up or seems overly sleepy or groggy in the morning, then it is a sign that they may not be getting sufficient sleep. Another sign that your older child is not getting enough sleep is if they quickly fall asleep throughout the day in situations where they would typically stay awake. Examples of this would be short car rides, watching a movie, reading a book, or doing homework. Other signs can be irritability, grumpiness, or behavior problems. One of the ways I monitor whether my children are getting enough sleep is by not using an alarm clock in their room. If they are not waking up naturally in the morning, they are not going to bed early enough at night and perhaps not getting adequate rest. If I have to wake them up to get ready for school, it indicates to me that I might need to move bedtime earlier. This may not work for all families, but you may want to consider giving it a try. It is also important to remember that sleep requirements change according to other factors such as stress, physical activity, travel, and illness. When my children are participating in intense sports, they often need more sleep. This also happens when they are recovering from illness. This is normal and should be expected.

Intuitive Sleeping?

Sleeping is similar to eating in many ways. Just like hunger, sleepiness comes with recognizable cues such as yawning, rubbing of the eyes, and having half-closed eyelids. Missing or ignoring these cues can lead to late signs of fatigue in babies and children, such as crying and tantrums, or behavior problems, such as aggression. Becoming sensitive to your child's sleepiness cues will help to foster healthy sleep habits for life.

Ways to Support Sleep in Your Child

Start supporting healthy sleep patterns for your child in infancy, but it is never too late to start. Remember that as a parent, you are the gatekeeper and the leader when it comes to protecting and supporting these healthy habits. It also benefits you to keep your child well-rested because they have fewer behavior problems, and it makes life easier and more enjoyable for everyone. But, ultimately, good sleep is relevant not just for the short-term but for long-term health.

Sleep hygiene refers to habits and practices that encourage good sleep. Just like we teach our children to brush their teeth and trim their nails, we can establish good habits related to ensuring that they sleep soundly and adequately.

1. **Have a regular sleep routine seven nights per week.** This may involve taking a warm bath, putting on pajamas, brushing teeth, and reading a book. Whatever routine you have, stick to it, and be consistent. Commitment and consistency to a regular sleep routine is key to healthy sleep patterns for the entire family.

2. **Go to sleep at the same time and wake up at the same time every day, not deviating more than one hour in either direction.** This is especially important for teens! When children reach adolescence, they may have a slight shift in their sleep schedule and lean toward a later bedtime; they may also be tempted to stay up very late on weekends. While it might seem that this is okay because they can "sleep in" the next morning, it actually disrupts sleep rhythms.

3. **Get exposure to sunshine early in the day.** Sunshine helps reinforce the circadian clock so that we are awake and sleepy at appropriate times.

4. **Ensure that your child is getting a minimum of thirty minutes of physical activity per day.** Adequate physical activity promotes better sleep.

5. **Avoid heavy meals right before bedtime.** Having too much food in the stomach can interrupt sleep cycles and make it harder to fall asleep. Try to end dinner at least two hours before bedtime.

6. **Start turning down lights in your house a couple of hours before bedtime.** Create a relaxing atmosphere in your home by playing soft music and diffusing essential oils, such as lavender. Decreasing light exposure in the evenings as the sun goes down also syncs our circadian rhythms. Some people are more sensitive to light than others and may be overly stimulated by light exposure in the evenings.

7. **Turn off and put away computers, smartphones, tablets, TVs, and other screens at least one hour before bedtime.** The light from screens tends to be a very bright light that stimulates our brains and activates wakefulness. Putting these devices away decreases our exposure and allows us to transition into activities that are more conducive to sleep.

a parent's guide to intuitive eating

8. Do not allow TVs or computers in your child's room. Multiple studies have shown that children who have televisions in their bedrooms sleep less and may have more nightmares and behavior problems. Having a TV in the room increases the likelihood that your child will stay up later than they should.

9. Keep rooms dark and cool. Use blackout shades and a fan as needed to keep rooms fresh. Minimize light exposure from electronics and other devices. Older kids can consider using a sleep mask to block out all light.

10. Use white noise. White noise machines block out noises and create a soothing blanket of sound to sleep to. We have used white noise machines in our house since my youngest was a newborn. However, you can also use a fan or an app on your phone or tablet. These apps are great for travel and come in particularly handy in hotels or other unfamiliar places where sleeping may be more difficult.

Signs of More Serious Sleep Problems

If you are practicing good sleep hygiene and your child is unable to sleep well, it might be time to seek professional help. Here are some signs that your child might be having more severe sleep problems:

1. Difficulty falling asleep. It should take no more than twenty minutes to fall asleep at night. If it regularly takes your child longer than this to fall asleep, talk to the doctor.

2. Waking up frequently throughout the night. If your child wakes up at night and has a difficult time falling back asleep on a recurrent basis, this can create chronic sleep deprivation.

3. Snoring or pauses in breathing during sleep. Sleep apnea is a medical condition in which a person experiences long pauses in their breathing at night. It can create short- and long-term health problems. If you notice your child snores heavily or has pauses in their breath at night, have them evaluated by a doctor.

4. Excessive daytime sleepiness, grogginess, or behavior problems. Even if you don't notice any of the above, but your child seems overly sleepy, groggy, grumpy, or has behavior problems, it could be caused by chronic sleep deprivation. Talk to your doctor if you are worried about this possibility.

Stress

Adults are often chronically exposed to stress, but we sometimes forget that our children might be experiencing stress too. Stress can come from many different areas of life. Tensions at home, difficulties with friendships, school, or work, demanding athletics, rigorous academics, or external pressures such as bullying can create stress for children.

What Is Stress?

In the simplest terms, stress is the body's reaction to a challenge resulting in physical, mental, or emotional responses. Stress can originate from many places, including our very own thoughts. When we feel stressed, physiological changes in our chemicals prepare us to react to the challenge. This is known as the "fight-or-flight" reaction in which our heart rate and blood pressure rise, our breathing changes, we get sweaty, and we become alert and prepared to make quick decisions. You may remember feeling these physiological changes if you've ever experienced stage fright or felt nervous before a test or interview. But not all stress is bad. Stress helps us stay safe and avoid danger. In fact, mild, infrequent stress can be healthy. It is when stress becomes frequent, severe, and chronic that it is no longer helpful and can lead to health problems.

How Chronic Stress Affects Our Metabolism and Eating Behaviors

Chronic stress leads to persistently elevated cortisol levels. Cortisol is a stress hormone that is necessary for human survival and optimal functioning of many organ systems. However, when it stays elevated, it can negatively affect our health because it affects metabolism. Besides affecting appetite and leading to overeating or undereating, stress can increase blood sugar levels, raise insulin, and cause insulin resistance, all while prompting children and adults to seek out foods that are high in fat and sugar. This is likely why chronic stress is associated with common chronic diseases such as diabetes and heart disease.

Other Consequences of Chronic Stress

Chronic stress creates generalized and nonspecific symptoms of disease such as diarrhea, upset stomach, indigestion, difficulty sleeping, difficulty concentrating, and headaches. It can lead to depression, anxiety, and panic attacks. Prolonged stress in children can even affect puberty, stature, and body composition. Children's developing brains may be more sensitive to the effects of stress than adults. Chronic stress can also trigger unhealthy compensatory addictive behaviors such as drug use, gambling, and overeating. Although these addictive behaviors are more common in adults, even young children can learn to use food as a soothing technique when they become overly stressed. Because of their increased independence, teenagers are at greater risk for drug abuse and dependence. Other signs of chronic stress in children include irritability, behavior problems, changes in sleep patterns, and changes in relationships or academic performance. As I mentioned in the sleep section, sleep deprivation leads to increases in the stress hormone cortisol, but chronic stress can also cause difficulty sleeping, which creates a double whammy.

Symptoms of chronic stress:

- Stomachaches
- Diarrhea
- Headaches
- Difficulty sleeping
- Anxiety
- Panic attacks

- Depression
- Irritability
- Behavior problems
- Overeating
- Engaging in too much screen time
- Social isolation

If you notice that your child has signs of chronic stress, the first thing to do is assess the situation and talk to your child about how they are feeling. When you speak to your child, validate their feelings and reassure them that it's okay and healthy to experience *all* emotions. If you believe that your child is overscheduled, evaluate this area. Can an activity be eliminated or put on hold for a while? What does your child like to do the most, and what is not as important? Keeping the lines of communication open with your child will help tremendously in this area. However, you can also teach your child healthy coping skills at home, which will be beneficial for life.

What Are Healthy Ways to Manage Stress?

Some stress is unavoidable in life, and some children will be more sensitive to stress or become anxious more quickly than others. Teaching children different ways to manage stress in healthy ways early on will benefit them for life.

1. Prayer, meditation, or quiet reflection. Taking fifteen to twenty minutes per day to sit quietly and reflect, pray, or meditate is ideal for all people, but it is especially important when one is experiencing stress.

2. Journaling. Journaling is an easy way to get thoughts out of our heads and onto paper, and some children may enjoy this. It is also inexpensive and can be done anywhere.

3. Exercise. There are physiological reasons why exercise fights stress and boosts mood. Even just going for gentle walks has psychological benefits. Many children also benefit from being out in nature.

4. Yoga or stretching. Yoga, stretching, and breathing exercises also promote relaxation.

5. Diffusing essential oils, such as lavender. Some essential oils can have a calming effect and have the added bonus of improving sleep. My favorite is lavender. Other oils known to have a stress-reducing effect include lemon, bergamot, ylang-ylang, and jasmine. Diffuse it or apply it to a sachet or pillowcase rather than applying it directly to the skin.

6. Talking it out with a friend or family. Sometimes when children are stressed, they may isolate themselves and avoid talking to other people. Children should have someone that they trust to talk to when they are feeling sad, anxious, and overwhelmed. It can be a family member or a trusted friend. Check in and make sure that your child feels that there is someone that they can talk to when they need help processing a challenge in their life.

When to Seek Help

If you feel that your child is overly stressed or anxious or has had a sudden or concerning change in behavior, please have them see a professional. An excellent place to start would be your pediatrician or family doctor, who can evaluate your child and may refer them to a counselor or therapist. A therapist can help your child learn different ways to think, which in turn helps decrease stress.

Exercise

Physical activity seems to come naturally to children. As soon as they can, children start to explore their environment by rolling, crawling, cruising, walking, running, and climbing. They can't seem to get enough and only stop at the end of the day when they pass out from exhaustion. Sometimes parents wish their kids would just sit still for a while, but it really is very healthy for children to be active.

Physical activity serves many functions. It strengthens bones and muscles, moves lymph fluid, helps return blood flow to the heart, and so much more. Research has found many benefits to exercise, including strengthened immunity, decreased risk of heart disease, and reduced risk of Alzheimer's disease. Staying active also improves sleep and positively affects metabolism. Exercise also has a beneficial influence on appetite-regulating hormones. Moderate exercise keeps joints healthy and decreases pain. Physically active people tend to have an easier time regulating their weight. The mental health benefits of exercise are amazing. Those who exercise regularly experience less anxiety and depression, and they sleep better too. My very favorite benefit of exercise and physical activity is my well-being. Being active just *feels* good. Kids intuitively know this. Movement is play, and play is movement. They do not see exercise as a way to "get in shape" or "burn calories." They just do it because it makes them happy. Adults tend to forget about the magic of movement over time and start seeing exercise as a chore or a punishment for the "sin" of eating chocolate cake.

How Physical Activity and Intuitive Eating Are Linked

In our society, we have started to associate exercise with weight loss or fitness. While physical activity can help people stabilize and regulate weight, linking the two can create unintended consequences. Studies show that people who exercise to "get in shape" are less likely to continue regular

a parent's guide to intuitive eating

exercise than people who exercise to feel good or because they wish to develop mastery. For those suffering from eating disorders, exercise can become a form of purging and it can feel like a punishing burden. The good news is that those who have strong intuitive eating skills are more likely to feel positively about exercise and those who are physically active are more likely to have healthy eating habits.

Changing Physical Activity Over Time

As I mentioned before, young children are naturally active and seem to be always on the go. However, this changes as they get older. By the time children get to middle school, they become more sedentary and they are spending more time sitting, watching television, and playing video games.

However, there are also personality differences when it comes to move-ment. My older son is a very high energy person and has a hard time sitting still. He thrives on lots of physical activity and really enjoys almost any physical challenge. My younger son is an expert "relaxer" and really enjoys his quiet time watching shows, reading, or playing video games. However, he LOVES sports and is particularly motivated by competition. Understanding that everybody has a different personality and different baseline energy levels is another way to honor the differences in our chil-dren. It also helps us find different ways to support and promote healthy physical activity in our children.

How to Support Healthy Physical Activity

Supporting physical activity is similar to promoting intuitive eating. To cre-ate a positive atmosphere for exercise and physical activity, set up habits and behaviors that you can model and do together as a family. However, there is no need to force physical activity. Just let it come naturally by cre-ating ample opportunities and creating an environment that promotes movement.

Here are some tips for integrating physical activity into your life and creating a lifelong habit in your children:

1. Make movement a part of your family life. A great way to help your child stay active is to integrate physical activity into your family lifestyle. In my family, we have started a Saturday hike, snowshoe outing, or other physical activity together. Although this does require more thought and planning, it is a great way to foster the love for movement and adventure.

2. Make your home a movement-friendly zone. When my oldest son was a toddler, I remember very clearly sitting in the middle of the living room floor, crying. One of my favorite clay pots was broken and I was grieving not being able to have any decorations. I made a decision that day to make life easier for my energetic toddler and me by shaping the environment around him. Removing all of the breakable and dangerous objects made it safe for him to be a kid and also decreased my stress level. As my kids grew, I continued this practice to support their natural desire to move. I kept the floors free of clutter and even purchased toys that could be used inside, such as plasma cars, bouncy toys, and mini trampolines. That way, they could have fun and be active all throughout the day, regardless of the weather. I also trained myself to be more tolerant of my children's need for movement and play. I can't say I am perfect at this, but I do my best. I let them run and play inside, but if they get too rowdy and I am feeling overwhelmed, I send them outside.

3. Model joyful movement. Find physical activities that you love and let your children see you enjoying them. Just like you can model intuitive eating of health-promoting foods, you can model the joy of moving your body.

4. Try new activities together. Be playful and adventurous. Have fun trying new sports and activities together as a family.

5. Support and encourage team and individual sports. Not all children enjoy team sports, but there are many solo sports to choose from, like cross country or track, swimming, tennis, and many more. Some children prefer team sports. There are advantages to both, and both can help children develop unique and valuable skills that can benefit them in other ways. It may take some time for children to find a sport they enjoy, so let them try different ones until they find the one that fits them best.

6. Create challenges and incentives. Some children are motivated by competition and reward. Wearing fitness tracking devices such as Fitbit can allow you to create family challenges that promote greater physical activity in your more competitive children. You can create a system in which children participate in physical activity to earn nonfood rewards such as media time.

Exercise and physical activity are essential components of a healthy lifestyle and support healthy eating. Finding ways to promote and encourage joyful movement in your family's life will help complement intuitive eating practices and create happy, healthy kids.

When you foster intuitive eating habits, offer health-promoting foods to your children, and promote the healthy lifestyle habits of sleep, exercise, and stress reduction, you will be giving your child the gift of a lifetime.

Chapter 9

Healthy Eating Habits

Now it's time to apply everything you've learned through the stages of growth, from pregnancy through high school. This is where I get into the nitty-gritty. Each phase brings different challenges and opportunities, and I will offer tips for various approaches to feed your developing child. Remember that you are growing and evolving along with your child, and the world also continues to change around you. That is why I encourage keeping a few concepts in mind that will help you be successful. First of all, what is success? In Chapter 1, I outlined three goals I have when I am feeding my children and my family. These are the same goals I have in mind when I provide you the advice in this book (see page 9).

I want kids to feel good, be free of preventable chronic disease, and be able to navigate the world of eating with ease all while possessing a positive body image. Note that nowhere did I say every kid will love broccoli and salad, avoid all processed foods, and have a "perfect" BMI. Why? Because achieving those things is not necessary for meeting the above goals.

What *is* necessary for success? First, let go of perfectionism. You don't have to be perfect (no one is!), just learn the skills and start practicing. Especially if these are new concepts to you, you will have to try them out and learn how to apply them to your life and your family through trial and error. Do the best you can and figure out what works for you. Let these skills and tools evolve with you and your family over time, and take a gentle approach.

Second, let go of fear. In my pediatric practice, I encounter a lot of scared parents. They are scared to make the wrong choices. They are afraid that their child is just not right nutritionally, developmentally, or medically. They fear that their child is too small or too big. Do you share any of these fears? Fear can be a beneficial emotion because it protects us from real danger, but in the modern world, we create fear from our own thoughts, and it can cause overanalysis without action, and an overwhelming urge to control. In terms of feeding our families, this toxic fear can lead to not making any changes at all, spending too much time, energy, and stress worrying about every single detail, or dedicating ourselves to controlling every morsel that crosses our children's mouths. To start practicing the principles of intuitive eating in your family, you must let go of fear. Trust your child, and trust that everything will be okay. There are situations where worry and concern are legitimate, and I will cover those in Chapter 17, Common Concerns. But for the most part, if your child is developing normally, growing along their curve, and thriving, let go of the fear and start practicing the skills.

Finally, I want you to believe that you are a good parent. Maybe you already do, and that is great—keep it up. I know a lot of parents have serious doubts. You may spend a lot of time guilting yourself or feeling guilted or shamed by family members or friends. Unfortunately, parenting is one of those areas where shaming has become very prevalent, and it's easy to start feeling like you aren't worthy of this role. Not only is this untrue, but pervasively feeling this way can be counterproductive to reaching your goals. Your children think you are terrific, and you are doing much better than you think. It can all feel so overwhelming and confusing. I know, I've been there. I am here to simplify it for you and to help you get there with less stress than before. What you believe you will embody. Believe in yourself, give yourself much-needed credit, and keep doing a great job. I believe in you and all that you do for your children and family.

Before you dive into each exciting stage of development, review and keep in mind The Five Pillars of Healthy Eating (see page 48).

A Word on Feeding Styles

The way that parents approach raising and feeding their children has been classified into categories. Most parents aren't all one way or another, but these are general patterns that some parents fall into. These parenting styles are not "good" or "bad," but one in particular—the authoritative feeding style—seems to be more conducive to intuitive eating and supporting children on a health-promoting eating journey. If you find yourself fitting into a less beneficial pattern for supporting intuitive eating, know that these styles are often learned from our own parents and might be passed down through generations. Instead of feeling guilty, pay attention to how you can start to shift these patterns closer to the authoritative feeding style.

Authoritarian Feeding Style

Parents who fall under this feeding style want to have as much control as possible over what their children eat. They control portions, may be more prone to urge their children to eat their vegetables, and use dessert as a bribe for eating their greens. Ironically, at least one study found that the authoritarian feeding style was associated with children eating *fewer* vegetables. These parents tend to set a lot of strict limits and have many rules. They limit what types of foods a child eats but also may force the child to eat foods they do not like. This leads to children not having a good sense of hunger and satiety and also not learning to trust themselves, their appetite, or their food choices.

Permissive/Indulgent Feeding Style

The permissive/indulgent parent style avoids conflict and wants to please their child. This leads to acting almost opposite to the authoritarian parent. The permissive parent has little rules and boundaries and tends to say "yes" to most requests. There may not be much structure for meals and snacks because the children are allowed to eat what they want throughout the day. These children may develop difficulties regulating their intake of foods.

Neglectful Feeding Style

The neglectful feeding style may occur when parents are rushed and busy or may not have the skills or experience necessary to plan, buy, or prepare appropriate foods. It can also arise when parents have little interest in food or eating. The availability of food may seem random and chaotic, and children may be expected to prepare their own meals from an early age. Again, there may not be much structure, but there is also not much consistency. These children may start to overfocus on food because it may be scarce and inconsistent.

Authoritative Feeding Style

Not to be confused with the authoritarian feeding style, *authoritative* feeding happens when parents set some boundaries but also allow their children the freedom to get to know their appetites and explore food. Authoritative parents trust their children while providing appropriate food and an environment conducive to healthy eating behaviors. Studies have found that the authoritative feeding style has the most beneficial effects and that authoritative parents are more likely to have fruits and vegetables available. Authoritative parents decide what and when to eat and allow their children to determine if and how much. However, they also set some boundaries that enable their children to learn the skills of intuitive eating in a safe and supported manner. For example, an authoritative parent will develop structure around meal and snack times instead of letting their child graze all day, encourage water drinking between meals instead of juice or caloric beverages, and ensure that their child is seated at the table to eat rather than eating in front of the television.

Reading this and the next section will teach you the basics of learning to be an authoritative feeder. Remember, you don't have to be perfect, but you do have to let go of fear and trust yourself and your child.

The Value of Your Time Investment

Planning and preparing nutritious and enjoyable meals for a family is time- and labor-intensive. With our busy modern lifestyles, it can feel like a heavy burden and unpleasant chore. However, it really pays to make this investment for your own health and the health of your family for years and decades to come. Those who spend more time preparing meals consume more fruits and vegetables, and spend less time eating out. If you are not already used to regularly preparing food for your family it may be daunting at first, but the more you practice, the smoother and more fun it will become. These habits pay off exponentially in the long run. When your children are small, enlist the help of your partner or other family members. As your children grow, they can start participating in the menu planning and preparation of the food that you will share together. I estimate that I spend about four hours per week planning, purchasing, and preparing meals for myself and my family. To me, this time is an invaluable investment in our health.

Learning to Cook

Learning to cook is a skill that takes practice, but you don't need to be afraid. Anybody can learn the basic skills of putting together a simple, nutritious meal.

In the resources section, I have listed several cookbooks that will help you start your journey. I will also provide a few very simple recipes throughout the next section of the book. However, if at first it feels overwhelming and time consuming, just hang in there—it gets easier with time and practice!

Don't shy away from using convenience items in your favor. Frozen fruits and vegetables, canned beans, and precooked, shelf-stable whole grains all save time. There are precut veggies, prewashed and cut greens and salad mixes. I still use a lot of these products because I value efficiency. After you get the hang of it, you may elect to purchase less convenience items to save money.

To get started with cooking you don't need much, just a simple kitchen setup, but once you know the basics, you may consider purchasing some very helpful kitchen appliances such as a good blender or food processor, a programmable pressure cooker, or a rice cooker. These appliances are not necessary for cooking healthful meals, but they can save time and effort.

Stocking Your Kitchen

When it comes to home food preparation, many thrive on ease and simplicity. Having ingredients for easy-to-prepare meals readily available in your pantry, refrigerator, and freezer will facilitate the habit of eating wholesome meals at home.

Family meals don't have to be gourmet. In fact, the simpler you keep things, especially at first, the more likely you are to stick with it.

Although this is not an exhaustive list, I have listed below some items that you can keep in your kitchen to support your family's healthy eating journey. This is meant to stimulate brainstorming. Feel free to exchange for fruits, vegetables, whole grains, legumes, and nuts that you and your family prefer in each category.

Countertop

- Apples
- Bananas

- Cherry tomatoes
- Mandarin oranges

Refrigerator

- Bell peppers
- Berries (strawberries, blueberries)
- Broccoli
- Cabbage
- Carrots (usually baby carrots)
- Corn tortillas
- Cucumber
- Garlic
- Ginger (I keep this in the freezer)
- Green onions
- Greens (kale, spinach, red lettuce)
- Herbs (cilantro, basil)
- Hummus
- Mushrooms
- Plant-based milk (oat, soy, hemp, cashew, flax, almond)
- Potatoes (sweet and regular)
- Tempeh
- Tofu
- Whole grain bread
- Whole grain flour tortillas

Pantry

- Barley
- Brown rice
- Brown rice cakes
- Canned beans
- Cooked, shelf-stable whole grains
- Diced tomatoes
- Dried legumes (black, pinto, navy, chickpeas, kidney, lentils, split peas)
- Dried unsweetened fruit (raisins, cranberries, dates)
- Onions (sweet and red)
- Polenta
- Popcorn
- Quinoa
- Raw seeds (flax, hemp, chia, sunflower, pumpkin)
- Raw unsalted nuts (cashews, almonds, walnuts)

a parent's guide to intuitive eating

- Rolled or steel cut oats

- Shelf-stable plant milk (oat, soy, hemp, cashew, flax, almond)

- Tomato paste

- Unsweetened applesauce

- Whole grain crackers

- Whole grain pasta

- Whole wheat couscous

Freezer

- Frozen fruit without added sweeteners (blueberries, strawberries, bananas, mangos, pineapple)

- Frozen precooked legumes (edamame, black-eyed peas)

- Frozen precooked whole grains (brown rice, quinoa)

- Frozen vegetables without added salt or oils (broccoli, green beans, sweet peas, sweet corn)

Condiments

- Apple cider vinegar

- Balsamic vinegar

- Dijon mustard

- Hot sauce

- Ketchup

- Miso paste (yellow or white)

- Mustard

- Salsa

- Seasoned rice vinegar

- Soy sauce or tamari

- Sriracha

- Vegetable bouillon or vegetable broth

Spices

- Chili powder
- Chipotle chili powder
- Cinnamon
- Cumin
- Curry powder
- Garlic powder
- Ginger
- Nutmeg
- Nutritional yeast
- Onion powder
- Oregano
- Paprika
- Sage
- Turmeric

Baking

- Baking powder
- Baking soda
- Dairy-free chocolate chips
- Cornmeal
- Cornstarch
- Ener-G egg replacer (or ground flaxseeds)
- Oat flour
- Pure maple syrup
- Silken tofu (Mori-Nu)
- Unsweetened cocoa powder
- Vanilla extract
- Whole wheat pastry flour

Creating Structure

I will go into each age group specifically in the next section, but once children are toddlers, it is beneficial to develop structure around meals and snacks. It is always important to be sensitive to your child's hunger and satiety cues; however, a general schedule is needed to establish a predictable routine that supports intuitive eating. This need not be rigid or inflexible. Create structure but allow it to bend and mold into your lifestyle. If structure is not created, there is a tendency for eating to become an all-day grazing session with one bite here and there or inconsistent and unplanned meals on the run. For example, in my family of two adults and two school-aged children, we tend to eat breakfast between 7 and 8 a.m., lunch from noon to 1 p.m., and dinner sometime between 4 and 6 p.m. After dinner, the kitchen is closed. My sons may or may not have an afternoon snack after school and this usually depends on what sports or activities they have that day. However, if everyone is hungry, we may elect to have dinner early instead. I like that my kids usually come to the dinner table hungry and ready to eat. If you have younger children, they may be eating more frequently so your schedule may look different.

The Power of Family Meals

Studies have found family meals to be a predictor of healthy children and teens. We live a busy, sometimes overscheduled life, which has led to eating on the run and fitting in food when we can. Unfortunately, this type of eating detracts from our efforts to help children learn the principles of intuitive eating. This is why I recommend the following default guidelines for eating. Obviously, they can't occur at every meal or every day. There must be some flexibility and adaptability, but the more you reinforce this eating pattern and routine, the better everyone in the family can tune into their bodies. I am very protective of these habits in my home because I know how quickly new patterns can develop.

1. Always eat sitting down. For children, this means sitting at a table or a high chair with a tray. Have a set location to eat meals, and keep it consistent. Avoid eating standing up, while walking around, in the car, and other places that are not ideal places to eat meals. It is helpful to keep the eating place primarily an eating place. Remove clutter and avoid doing stressful work at the table. If the table is piled high with books and papers, you will be less likely to sit there to eat a relaxed and enjoyable meal together.

2. Avoid distractions. Turn off the television, put away phones, tablets, and computers, and avoid loud, distracting music when eating. We are so used to multitasking that many people feel uncomfortable just eating and doing nothing else. However, this detracts from our ability to tune in and notice our signals of hunger and fullness. Regularly eating while watching television, reading, or texting leads to mindless eating. Besides, it steals from the pleasure of eating! This includes doing homework. I prefer my children have their snack and then do their homework separately. This leads to more mindful eating and more mindful homework completion.

3. Keep meals calm, relaxed, and pleasant. Make sure to set aside enough time so that you aren't feeling rushed or stressed. Avoid stressful conversations at dinnertime. Also, plan meals so that you have plenty of time to eat and finish before moving on to the next activity.

4. Tune into and enjoy your meal. When you sit back, relax, and enjoy your meal and the sensations in your body, you are role modeling this behavior to your children and family. It's a win-win situation.

Little Eyes Are Always Watching

One of the most important things that you can do as a parent is to model the behaviors that you would like to pass on to your children. It may seem like they aren't paying attention, but studies show that children tend to follow suit of their parents, and it starts earlier than you may even think. A mother's lifestyle choices, including exercise and alcohol consumption, can predict the weight status of her offspring. Little eyes are always observing their surroundings. If you feel that your eating habits need improvement, it might be time to start easing yourself into some new habits. This applies to eating intuitively and eating health-promoting foods. It doesn't have to be all-or-nothing, but it is going to be tough to expect your child to taste and explore new foods if you display a restrictive eating style yourself. Remember, it's never too early or too late to start.

Firing the Food Police

The moralization of the health benefits or detriments of food can undermine intuitive eating. It's one thing to learn about how foods can help or harm us, but it is quite another to believe that eating a certain way is inherently wrong. As parents, we have to make many choices in raising our children and keeping them safe and healthy. Sometimes it is easier to make things black and white. For some things in life, such as never running across a parking lot or never opening the door to a stranger, this approach works. But using absolute rules and fear-based tactics for food can lead to greater troubles. Fear often leads us to draw lines in the sand. We are afraid that if our children eat and like donuts, they may never eat a vegetable again. Even if we aren't explicit about these moralizations, they come out in subtle ways. A typical example is to call all processed foods "junk food." This may seem harmless, but it is one method we use in our society to discourage a particular choice.

It may seem like it would be easier to categorize all foods into "good" or "bad." However, this often backfires. It leads to children that rebel and indulge only in the so-called "bad" foods or become obsessed with perfection and avoid all "bad" foods at any cost. It can lead to judgment and moralizing of other people's food decisions as well. Some people may start to believe that if they eat or desire "bad" foods, then they are wrong or damaged themselves. Moralizing food hurts us. There exists so much guilt and shame surrounding food but this is simply unnecessary. The truth is no food is all good or all bad. Food is food. Food is *neutral*. As I described in the previous section, there are potential benefits and potential harms, but these are not absolute. The most health-promoting path is that which follows a general pattern that emphasizes those foods that have more benefits.

How you discuss food is one of the hardest obstacles to navigate in your family's intuitive eating journey. How will you approach situations in which your child reaches for food that makes you feel uncomfortable? You may experience a myriad of feelings from fear that they will be unhealthy, gain weight, or that you will be judged for being a bad mom because you let your child eat a donut. What is most important to me is ensuring that I do not convey to my little one that there is something wrong or bad about them because they chose and ate that food. Instead of moralizing, let's normalize. Let's talk about how these foods really do call out to us, and they really do taste delicious. Instead of feeling bad about wanting these foods, let's shift the conversation to how we can balance these types of foods in an overall health-promoting pattern of eating that is enjoyable and sustainable for a lifetime.

By now you should feel comfortable with techniques that you can employ to support and encourage intuitive and health-promoting eating in your home. Finally, it is time to explore each unique and exciting stage in development and how you can apply these skills along the way!

part IV

Feeding Your Child through the Years

"The early years are when you give your child a foundation for establishing a proper diet. If kids learn about the importance of eating healthy early in their lives, they will not have to relearn as an adult."

—Nicole Henderson, CEO of Selsi Enterprises

Chapter 10

Pregnancy:
Preparing Yourself and Your Baby for an Intuitive Eating Journey

I f you are reading this book while you are pregnant or before you conceive, congratulations! Pregnancy is such a special time! You are anticipating the arrival of your little one, imagining what he or she will look like, and dreaming about all the fun you will have together in the years to come. But you also are indulging in treats and pampering yourself as you await your bundle of joy. During pregnancy, women carrying a single baby require about 300 extra calories per day, so you really do need a little extra energy intake. However, this is also one of the most valuable times in your life to focus on eating health-promoting foods. You are no longer just feeding yourself. You and your baby share the exact same blood! You are supplying 100 percent of the oxygen, vitamins, and nutrients that your baby needs to grow and develop. Believe it or not, your baby actually starts TASTING in the womb! By eight weeks of gestation, neural tracts have emerged in the brain that will allow your baby to differentiate between sweet, salty, sour, bitter, and umami. However, fetuses don't actually start swallowing and tasting until sixteen weeks when taste buds form. By twenty-one weeks, they are swallowing several ounces of amniotic fluid per day! This means that even before your baby is born, you can start to shape and influence their taste preferences. This is incredibly powerful! If you expose your growing baby to fruits, vegetables, whole grains, beans, nuts, and seeds now, they are more likely to accept these types of foods later. Also, when you eat a variety of whole plant foods, you are consuming vitamins and nutrients that are necessary to grow a healthy baby.

Folic acid is required for the proper development of the spinal cord and nervous system in babies. In fact, folic acid is so vital that in the United States food companies started fortifying many processed foods with this vitamin in 1998 to protect the public. Your prenatal vitamin supplies sufficient folic acid. However, folic acid is also naturally abundant in leafy greens, which are also rich in calcium, iron, and other nutrients that are vital for pregnant mamas to consume. Legumes are another great source of iron and calcium, and a denser source of calories and protein.

A diet high in fiber will aid digestion and keep you regular. Constipation is a common side effect of pregnancy. Eating whole plant foods can help ease this common complaint.

It is advisable to take a prenatal multivitamin during your pregnancy. I recommend Dr. Fuhrman's gentle prenatal if you don't already have a recommendation from your doctor. Fully plant-based or vegan mothers should take special care to supplement their vitamin B12 during pregnancy and while breastfeeding. There is also mixed evidence that taking an omega-3 fatty acid supplement with DHA and EPA may benefit your baby.

Foods to avoid during pregnancy include the following:

- **Alcohol.** There is no known safe amount of alcohol consumption during pregnancy, so it is best to avoid it altogether.

- **Caffeine.** It is wise to limit caffeine, although a cup or two of coffee per day is unlikely to cause harm. The same is true with herbal teas.

- **Raw meats, processed meats, and raw dairy.** These carry a high risk of infection that could be dangerous during pregnancy. Additionally, avoid large predator fish such as swordfish, shark, tilefish, and king mackerel as they are more likely to contain dangerous levels of mercury, which can harm your baby.

Also, make sure to check with your doctor before you take any medications or supplements as they could affect your baby.

Pregnancy Power Foods

Vegetables: Leafy greens such as kale, broccoli, and spinach are exceptional sources of calcium, iron, and folic acid. It may be easier for some pregnant women who can't handle volume to consume them in smoothies, puree them into sauces, or cook them into soups.

Fruits: Naturally sweet and satisfying, fruits are a great way to tackle that sweet tooth but also provide antioxidants and beneficial vitamins.

Beans: Beans, lentils, and split peas are packed with fiber, antioxidants, protein, and complex carbohydrates. They contain calcium and iron and are also one of the top sources of folic acid. Beans are a great way to bulk up your meals if you need a calorie boost and can also help you stay regular if you are suffering from constipation.

Whole grains: Brown rice, quinoa, and oatmeal are all fantastic sources of complex carbohydrates, fiber, and nutrients. Eating oats in the postpartum period may help some mothers produce more breast milk.

Nuts and seeds: Another way to bulk up calories for women who are only able to get in small meals toward the end of pregnancy, nuts are delicious and contain selenium, zinc, and folic acid. Walnuts, hemp seeds, chia seeds, and ground flaxseeds are also a good source of plant-based omega-3 fatty acids.

When you take care of your own health and nutrition during pregnancy, you are also taking care of your unborn baby. Start practicing these habits early on so that it is easier to continue the trend in the following stages of growth.

Morning Sickness

Ninety percent of pregnant women experience some degree of nausea and vomiting during pregnancy. Most develop it within the first two months and have relief by four to five months of gestation. The majority of women will have only mild symptoms, but some women may experience nausea and vomiting so severe that it seriously interferes with their health and quality of life. Because of this, many women may experience difficulty eating vegetables during the early months of their pregnancy. If this is the case for you, let go of any guilt and do the best you can. You will feel better eventually, and when you do, you can proceed to include back those foods that may currently disgust you. In the meantime, focus on eating what whole foods you *can* tolerate, eat small meals, and don't neglect your vitamins! Keep meals simple and have healthful options easily accessible and within view. If you enjoy smoothies, I have included a couple of easy recipes in this chapter that contain powerful antioxidants and iron-rich leafy greens.

Popeye Smoothie

Simple, creamy, and delicious! A fantastic way to get a full serving of leafy greens with naturally sweet fruit.

Serves: 1 to 2

1 cup soy, almond, cashew, coconut, or oat milk

2 pitted Medjool dates or 1 cup chopped green fruits such as apple, kiwi, or pears

1 frozen banana

1 cup spinach or kale

Add all ingredients to the blender and blend until smooth. Enjoy!

Dr. Yami's Super Antioxidant Smoothie

This recipe includes greens, berries, herbs, and spices, all of which are packed with antioxidants. If you are experiencing nausea, consider adding fresh or ground ginger.

Serves: 1 to 2

1 (15-ounce) can pears in juice

1 cup seedless red grapes

4 mint leaves

½ teaspoon ground turmeric

2 large handfuls spinach or kale

1 frozen banana

1½ cups frozen mixed berries

Add all ingredients to the blender and blend until smooth. Enjoy.

Body Image during Pregnancy

The body changes significantly during pregnancy to support and accommodate a growing baby. Some women find pregnancy liberating and develop a love and appreciation of their bodies. Other women may mourn the changes in their bodies and have a harder time with the transition.

Pregnancy is the perfect time to start practicing the principles of intuitive eating. It is not a time to diet or attempt to restrict calories. This can cause growth restriction and low birth weight in your baby. It is also an excellent time to start practicing body respect and appreciation. Instead of focusing on the changes in your shape, shift your thoughts to how impressive it is that your body is growing a baby! It truly is awe-inspiring and fascinating.

Here are a few more tips to improve your body image and find support during this unique and vulnerable period:

1. Surround yourself with support. Don't be afraid to be honest about your feelings and fears. You'll likely be surprised by how many other women have felt precisely the same way you do.

2. Stay active. Choose physical activities that feel good. Walking and swimming are low-impact activities that you can continue throughout your pregnancy. Make sure you discuss with your health-care provider what exercises are appropriate for you during your pregnancy.

3. Be nourished. Eat meals that satisfy you and give you energy. Tune into your body and trust your hunger and fullness.

4. Practice self-care. This can be as simple as giving yourself permission to take a much-needed nap or allowing time to meditate or journal your feelings.

5. Seek help. If you are struggling, talk to your OB/GYN or find a trusted therapist. Pregnancy and the postpartum period can be difficult for some women who may suffer from depression or anxiety. Seeking help is not a sign of weakness. Finding support when you need it is healthy for you and your baby and can help you develop the skills and tools to feel healthy and empowered for your family.

Vegan Whole Wheat Waffles

Enough to satisfy your cravings, but wholesome and packed with fiber. Top with plenty of fruits and dig in!

Serves: 4 to 6

2 tablespoons ground flaxseed meal	2 to 3 cups plant-based milk, such as almond, soy, coconut, or oat
3 tablespoons water	½ teaspoon salt
2 cups whole wheat flour	1 cup raw walnuts, chopped
4 teaspoons baking powder	

1. Preheat waffle iron.

2. Whisk ground flaxseed meal with 3 tablespoons of water until it thickens. This is your flax "egg."

3. Mix the whole wheat flour, baking powder, plant-based milk, flax egg, and salt in a medium bowl. Fold in the walnuts. The waffle mix should be thick but not too thick to create fluffy and crispy waffles.

4. Spray the waffle iron with a nonstick spray. Spread the waffle mix on waffle iron and cook according to waffle iron specifications.

Topping suggestions: strawberries, blueberries, bananas, nut butter, maple syrup

Key Points

- Emphasize health-promoting whole plant foods during your pregnancy, including an abundance of fruits, vegetables, whole grains, beans, nuts, and seeds.

- If you aren't already an intuitive eater, practice tuning into your body and recognizing your hunger and fullness signals.

- Take your prenatal vitamin and consider taking a vegan omega-3 DHA/EPA supplement if it's okay with your doctor.

- Enjoy your changing pregnant body and stay active in ways that feel good.

- Dieting during pregnancy can harm your baby but can also prevent you from practicing the principles of intuitive eating. If you feel the need to diet, reach out for support.

- Anxiety and depression can affect some women during pregnancy and in the postpartum period. Get help as soon as possible for the benefit of yourself and your baby.

Chapter 11

Early Infancy and Lactation: Newborn through 6 Months

O nce your baby is born, the real fun begins! The journey of feeding starts right after birth with the big decision of whether or not you will choose to provide your baby with your own milk. Although breastfeeding affords you and your child a host of benefits, not all mamas may have the opportunity to nurse their babies. If you adopted your child or you have medical complications that prevent breastfeeding, you may not be able to nurse your baby. This can be emotionally burdensome for some mothers but know that plenty of babies have been raised on formula (me!), and they do just fine. There are also many moms who choose both breast milk and formula or exclusively formula from the beginning for a variety of reasons.

Development and Characteristics

Full-term babies are born with an intact suck-and-swallow reflex that allows them to latch onto a breast and suckle instinctively. In the first few weeks of life, babies spend most of their time sleeping, eating, and digesting. During this time, they are rapidly growing and developing. Babies usually double their birth weight by six months of age and triple their weight by twelve months of age! Their brain cells are proliferating as they learn all about the world around them. Even though babies are born with the instinct to show hunger cues, you still have to interpret and react to these signs. It's like learning to dance with your baby.

Whether you breastfeed, bottle-feed, or formula-feed your baby, it is imperative to start to recognize, be sensitive to, and respond to their hunger and satiety cues. Each baby is different, but there are some common hunger cues that babies display. Although we typically think of crying as the way that babies communicate, it is actually a late cue, which means that most babies actually show other more subtle signs that they are hungry *before* they progress to crying as a last resort. These subtle signs are called early hunger cues. In the beginning, you may miss these signs until you get to know your baby better, but don't fret, you'll get plenty of practice as the days and weeks pass.

Hunger cues in newborns and young infants:

- Opening and closing the mouth

- Stirring and becoming restless

- Sucking on lips and tongue

- Sucking on hands

- Rooting (This is a motion where the mouth and head move back and forth as if seeking a nipple.)

- Crying

Satiety cues in newborns and young infants:

- Falling asleep

- Slowing down in suck-and-swallow rate

- Dropping off from the nipple

- Pursing lips and turning away

- Arching back and pushing away

How to Feed Your Infant

Breastfed Babies

If you choose to nurse your baby, you will continue to require extra calories, usually 300 to 400 extra calories per day for a single baby. Breastfeeding can be tough initially, but once you and your baby get the hang of it, it is a great way to bond and feed your newborn milk that was created especially for them. Breast milk has some amazing benefits. For mothers, breast-feeding helps tighten up the uterus and decreases the risk of hemorrhage after birth. It also reduces the risk of ovarian and breast cancer. Breast milk is often gentler on the baby's tummy, provides the perfect mix of macro-nutrients, contains maternal antibodies so that the baby acquires passive immunity and has less risk of infections, and may be associated with higher IQ later in life. Plus, it can save you money and is very convenient!

Breast milk tastes fantastic to babies, but in addition to that, it is another great way to start exposing your baby to the flavors of health-promoting foods like vegetables, fruits, and legumes. Amazingly, babies can taste the flavors of the foods you eat through your breast milk. This makes it worth-while to continue to eat health-promoting foods while you nurse your baby. If you are a nursing mother, continue to eat plenty of vegetables, fruits, beans, nuts, and seeds. You will provide the flavors of these foods to your baby through your breast milk in addition to the vitamins and nutrients that are health-promoting for you and your baby. Breastfed babies are less likely to be picky eaters and are more willing to try new foods when they are older.

Continue to take your prenatal vitamin for the entirety of your time nursing. Fully plant-based and vegan moms should also continue to supplement B12. Breast milk is naturally low in vitamin D. If you want to supplement your baby's vitamin D through your own milk, make sure you are taking at least 6,400 IU per day. Otherwise, breastfed babies require daily vitamin D supplementation of at least 400 IUs per day.

After birth and in their first few weeks, babies should be offered the breast at least every two to three hours throughout the day and night. Follow your baby's cues. In the first few days after birth, mothers produce a thick substance called colostrum. It usually takes two to four days for mother's full milk to come in. Before the milk is in, babies may seek the breast more frequently than every two to three hours. This actually helps stimulate your milk production. However, if you start to get too sore, make sure that your baby has established an appropriate latch and you are reinforcing good latching habits from the beginning.

Learning how to nurse your baby can be a nerve-wracking process. Even though it is a "natural" process, both you and your baby have to learn to do something you have never done before. Although persistent difficulties don't occur to the majority of mamas, there can be little bumps in the road. In addition to improper latch, tongue tie and a low milk supply can occur and can be very frustrating and disheartening for moms. It is never too early to seek the assistance of an experienced nurse, midwife, lactation consultant, or breastfeeding support group such as La Leche League if you are having difficulty.

As babies grow, they may sleep for longer stretches at night, which is usually great news for tired moms and dads. There are times that babies will cluster feed during growth spurts, meaning that they will eat more frequently.

This is an indication that their appetite is increasing temporarily. If baby displays early hunger cues, responding at that time will help support their intuitive eating skills. It is also helpful to avoid using the breast to calm the baby in every time of distress. If you are unsure if your baby is truly hungry, you can try other soothing techniques first such as swaddling, shushing, swinging, and sucking. I really love how these techniques are described and demonstrated in *The Happiest Baby on the Block* book and videos.

You will visit your baby's pediatrician within the first two weeks to ensure proper weight gain, but if you have concerns before that visit, don't hesitate to call the doctor. Unless your doctor recommends that you have a home scale for some reason, don't weigh your baby at home on a regular basis. This can be unnecessarily anxiety-provoking for many parents.

How long to breastfeed your child is up to you. The American Academy of Pediatrics recommends a minimum of six months of exclusive breastfeeding, and the World Health Organization recommends at least twelve months. I am thrilled when my patients are breastfed until a year of age. Many children will naturally wean from the breast between eighteen months and twenty-four months, but some children are nursed longer.

Going back to work might present an obstacle for some mothers. To maintain a milk supply, working mothers must continue to pump milk on the same schedule that their babies are feeding. Because babies fed breast milk or formula via bottle sometimes end up taking in a greater volume, it can be challenging for some mothers to keep up. Any breast milk is better than no breast milk. Even if you can't supply all of your baby's milk, do as much as you can, as long as you are willing.

I had my oldest son when I was in medical school. I felt lucky to have been able to nurse him until he was six months old, but around that point, finding time to pump during busy and stressful rotations was very challenging, and I weaned him. Thankfully he has grown into a handsome and healthy boy. It can be very emotional, but just know that whatever you choose, your baby will be okay.

Bottle- and Formula-Fed Babies

Between birth and six months of age, your baby requires only breast milk or infant formula. As far as I know at this time, fully plant-based formula is not available on the market. For those who want to avoid cow's milk–based formula, I recommend a soy formula or a hydrolyzed formula such as Nutramigen or Alimentum. A hydrolyzed formula breaks down the milk proteins so that they are less likely to cause a reaction in babies, especially those that might have an allergy or sensitivity to cow's milk protein. All of these can be purchased at your local pharmacy or grocery store. If you have already started your baby on a traditional formula and they are doing well, continue the same formula through twelve months of age.

Some parents may have heard that soy formula has potentially harmful effects, but a meta-analysis of thirty-five studies of soy infant formula found no significant differences in babies fed soy formula compared to babies fed conventional formula or breast milk in terms of growth, bone health, or metabolic, reproductive, endocrine, immune, and neurological functions.

If you choose to formula-feed your baby from birth, start low and go slow. Right after birth, babies do not need a large volume of milk. Their bodies and tummies are adjusting to being outside the womb, and they often spit up amniotic fluid in the first twenty-four hours. Start with 20 to 30 ml of milk every two to three hours. By two days of age, they are usually taking 30 to 60 ml every two to three hours.

Just like breastfed babies, formula-fed babies will display signs of hunger, and it is preferable to feed on demand by learning and following your baby's hunger signals. Formula-fed babies are a little more likely to be overfed than breastfed babies because we prepare a predetermined amount of formula and often expect the baby to finish the entire bottle. Fluids are delivered more quickly through a bottle than breast milk does through nursing, so satiety signals may lag. Bottle-fed babies tend to finish

a parent's guide to intuitive eating

eating faster than breastfed babies, which may lead to missed satiety cues. Using slow-flow nipples might help prevent babies from guzzling milk.

The volume of milk that a bottle-fed baby consumes will increase over time. But like all things, the amount each baby takes will be a bit different based on their size, age, and genetic differences. Bottle-fed babies will also experience growth spurts in which they suddenly demand more milk. Below are the general ranges for the amount of formula babies tend to consume at different ages.

Formula-Feeding Guide

0 TO 2 DAYS	1 to 2 oz every 2 to 3 hours
3 DAYS TO 2 WEEKS	2 to 3 oz every 2 to 4 hours
3 WEEKS TO 2 MONTHS	2 to 4 oz every 3 to 4 hours
3 TO 5 MONTHS	4 to 7 oz 5 to 6 times per day
6 TO 9 MONTHS	4 to 8 oz 4 to 6 times per day
10 TO 12 MONTHS	6 to 8 oz 4 to 6 times per day

When bottle-feeding, make sure you are following these safety guidelines:

1. Avoid homemade formulas. These are generally unsafe. Unless your child has food allergies/sensitivities *and* you are under the care of a dietitian who can ensure that the formula is safe, homemade formulas can lead to growth problems and nutrient deficiencies. Do not use store-bought cow's milk or plant-based milk for children under one year of age. The calorie content is too low, it is not fortified with sufficient vitamins, and it can cause other medical problems.

2. Never dilute your baby's formula. Powdered formula or premixed formula is intended to have a certain number of calories and is perfectly balanced for your baby's bloodstream. Diluting formula can lead to undernutrition and can cause dangerous shifts in the electrolytes in your baby's blood, which can lead to seizures and even death.

3. Do not prop your baby's bottle. It is tempting to prop a bottle when you are busy and have many other things to do. But this makes it very difficult to respond to your baby's satiety signals and may lead to overfeeding.

4. Never let a baby go to bed with a bottle. When babies get older and hold the bottle themselves, some parents are tempted to put baby to bed with a bottle so that they fall asleep on their own. This can increase the risk of ear infections and cavities and reinforces the habit of eating to go to sleep.

Fostering Intuitive Eating in Your Infant

When your baby is small and feeding exclusively on breast milk or formula, supporting intuitive eating is simple. Feed on demand based on your infant's hunger cues to best develop trust, establish a habit of eating for hunger, and establish stopping at satiety.

Babies don't need to be fed at every sign of discomfort or distress. This may set up the habit of feeding to self-soothe. Although breastfed babies may seek the breast to self-soothe as well as eat, bottle-fed babies can be at risk of overfeeding if they are offered a bottle at every peep. If this occurs frequently, it can contribute to a learned association.

Another area of trouble is ignoring when babies are full and coaxing them to continue to eat. This is more common with bottle-feeding, and also more likely to occur if parents or other family members are concerned about growth or weight gain.

Besides these two areas, once you develop a routine and flow with your baby, your job is to recognize and respond to cues. Your baby will decide when she has had enough.

Special Considerations

Infant Colic

Few things are more stressful than an angry, crying baby that cannot be consoled.

Unfortunately, this is the case with colic, which can be very trying for parents. Colic is defined as crying for no apparent reason for at least three hours per day at least three days a week in an otherwise healthy, typically developing baby that is less than three months old. These episodes tend to cluster in the evening. Colic develops during the first few weeks of life. Although researchers are still not certain what causes colic, for colicky breastfed babies, one of the first things that I do is have mom completely eliminate dairy from her diet. This includes milk, yogurt, cheese, ice cream, or anything that lists dairy in the first three ingredients.

Dairy has many names. Look for the following terms on food labels: milk, butter, cream, cheese, curds, casein, caseinate, whey, ghee, lactalbumin, or lactulose. Soy is another protein that crosses into the breast milk and may contribute to sensitivities in babies, and it is estimated up to 50 percent of babies who are sensitive to cow's milk protein will also react to soy protein.

Cow's milk protein intolerance or sensitivity can occur in 1 to 2 percent of babies. It is a medical condition in which the baby's gut reacts to a protein in cow's milk. It can occur in both breastfed and formula-fed babies. The typical symptoms I see are fussiness and colic, spitting up, diarrhea, and sometimes, bloody stools. Some babies are exquisitely sensitive and may have visible blood in their stool after their mother has even one exposure to dairy. The good news is that most babies tend to outgrow this by nine months of age. For formula-fed babies that are consuming a cow's milk–based formula and have symptoms of cow's milk protein intolerance, it might be reasonable to try a hydrolyzed formula like Nutramigen or Alimentum to see if symptoms resolve.

Key Points

- Become familiar with and respond to your baby's hunger and satiety cues.

- If you choose to nurse, continue to eat an abundance of vegetables, fruits, whole grains, beans, and nuts and seeds as this will continue to influence your baby's future taste preferences.

- Bottle-fed infants tend to eat faster than breastfed babies. Pay attention to satiety signals to avoid overfeeding. Avoid using milk to soothe your baby when they are not hungry.

- Never force a baby to eat past fullness.

- Breastfed and formula-fed babies can develop intolerances and sensitivities. If your baby develops vomiting, diarrhea, or blood in their stools, see a medical provider immediately.

Chapter 12

First Foods:
6 Months through 1 Year

B y around six months of age, babies can roll over and sit up, supported. They start reaching out for objects (including their feet!) and bringing them to their mouths. They have usually doubled their weight by six months. Some babies are considerably plump by this age. This is very normal! Sitting up on their own and crawling does not usually occur until eight or nine months of age. Many babies start cruising on furniture at around ten months. This change in activity level may slightly affect the weight velocity of some babies, especially if they are breastfed. Babies also rapidly develop in their social interactions. They are now playing, laughing, babbling, and imitating facial expressions.

By six months of age, your baby will be ready for solids! This is such a fun time! Prepare for funny faces, laughter, and dirty floors. Although I encourage mothers to exclusively breastfeed for at least four to six months, I recommend waiting no later than six months to introduce solids in a baby who was born full term (greater than thirty-eight weeks gestation). Waiting longer than six months increases the risk of developing food allergies, and of missing the critical window, you have to introduce stronger flavors of some health-promoting foods, such as bitter vegetables. However, do not start solids before four months of age because that can also increase the risk of allergies and other medical problems. Also, do not start solids at any age with the intent of helping your baby sleep longer at night if they are not showing signs of readiness.

Signs of readiness for solids:

- Sits up well, supported or on their own

- Seems interested (often mesmerized) in food and will reach out for it

- Opens mouth for food

- Able to swallow food (has lost the tongue-thrust reflex and no longer pushes out most food)

Transitioning to Solids

When you first start offering your baby complementary foods, they are intended to be part of the developmental process and will contribute very little to caloric intake. Have fun and don't stress about it. The primary source of nutrition for your baby is still going to be breast milk or formula for the first twelve months of life. Despite starting solids, the amount of breast milk or formula a baby eats should not significantly decrease until they are closer to one year of age.

In the United States, rice cereal mixed with either breast milk or formula has traditionally been a preferred first food. The rationale is that rice is less likely to trigger food allergies or reactions. However, oatmeal or another whole grain cereal also works well as a first food. That first week of rice cereal or oatmeal is a great way to test readiness and get them familiar with eating solids. Another advantage of feeding cereals, however, is that they are often iron-fortified and can provide a source of iron for breastfed babies.

When you first start to offer solids, feed your baby just once per day, preferably after they have received some breast milk or formula. Feed your baby sitting up in a high chair and with a spoon. If your baby still has the tongue-thrust reflex, he may not be ready. You will know this is the case because the majority of what you put in will come right back out. Try again in another week or two. Do not put rice cereal in your baby's bottle unless you are instructed to do so by your pediatrician.

After a baby does well with cereal once a day for a week or so, I suggest that you move on to green vegetables. There is evidence that babies are more receptive to stronger flavors during a small window of opportunity between four and seven months of age. During this time, they are more likely to accept these flavors and come to prefer them. I recommend that parents introduce green vegetables as soon as possible. You can make your own or select baby foods that consist of a single ingredient and have no added sugar or salt. Teach your baby to learn to enjoy the authentic flavors of food without enhancements. For the first few weeks after starting solids, wait at least three days in between new foods so that you can isolate for food allergies or reactions. Experiment with a greater variety of fruits and veggies and different types of whole grains. Babies learn to accept different flavors through variety and repeated exposure. Don't be surprised or discouraged if your baby grimaces and makes dramatic facial expressions when tasting new foods! This is normal and not a reason to stop offering the food.

Introduce Peanut Butter Early

A newer recommendation is to introduce peanut butter to babies after six months of age. You can either give some thinned with water or mix a bit of it in their cereal or fruit. The latest research shows that the early introduction of peanut butter actually helps to decrease the risk of peanut allergy, especially for babies that have eczema or an egg allergy.

Introduce legumes after your baby has established a good foundation of vegetables, fruits, and whole grains for about a month and is at least six months of age. Beans, lentils, and split peas are a great source of iron, calcium, and antioxidants, and it pays to familiarize your baby with these flavors early on. Iron is especially important for breastfed babies as breast milk is naturally low in iron and their iron stores may start to decrease by six months of age. Start with smaller legumes such as lentils and split peas, which are easier to digest. You can then move on to the larger beans, ensuring that they are well-cooked, soft, and pureed or mashed.

By nine months of age, babies will be eating solids twice per day, and by twelve months of age, they should be eating solids three times per day with snacks, as needed.

By nine months of age, most babies are ready for finger foods, although some may be ready before then. Watch for signs of readiness for self-feeding, and don't be afraid to let your baby transition to feeding them-selves. This is fun because they can explore a wider array of food textures and have more control over how much they eat.

Keep It Whole

Stick with whole foods as much as possible when feeding your baby. An incredible variety of fruits, vegetables, legumes, whole grains, and nut and seed butters is available to offer your baby. Tons of convenience products are on the market now, including puffs and crackers. However, these are all processed foods that are low in fiber and antioxidants. Although they may seem fun and made specifically for babies, remember that feeding babies is a business and getting parents to believe that they need to buy their babies special "baby foods" is a great way to make money. Use these foods sparingly.

Fabulous finger foods include pieces of soft fruit such as bananas and avo-cados, cooked veggies such as carrots, green beans, broccoli, well-cooked mashed beans, and soft whole grain pasta. Always feed your child while they are sitting up in a high chair, and avoid giving them too many foods

a parent's guide to intuitive eating

at once. One to two foods on their high chair tray is enough for them to explore and play with.

> ## Rescue Maneuvers for a Choking Baby
>
> If your baby appears to be choking and is unable to clear their airway, first open their mouth. If you can see the food, draw it out with your finger by gently sweeping it toward yourself. However, if they have a weak or absent cry or seem to have difficulty breathing, you may need to perform back blows and chest thrusts to expel the food item. If someone is around, have them call 911 while you start the maneuvers. First, gently turn your baby onto their stomach on your forearm as you cradle their chin in your hand and position the head lower than their chest. Then, deliver four firm blows between the shoulder blades with the heel of your hand. You then turn the baby over on your forearm onto their back (head still below chest) and deliver five chest thrusts with two to three fingers at the breastbone just below the nipple line at the center of the chest. You should compress about one-and-a-half inches. You keep repeating these maneuvers until the object is expelled. You can find guides with images at redcross.org.

By the time they are twelve months old, your baby will be eating three meals per day with snacks. By this age, most babies are eating what their family eats at each mealtime. Focus on a health-promoting menu that will benefit *everyone* in the household.

Baby-Led Weaning

Baby-led weaning is an alternative approach to feeding children that has become more popular recently. Weaning, in this case, does not mean weaning from the breast or bottle, it is a term used in the UK for introducing solid foods. In baby-led weaning, you let the baby take the lead on which foods he or she will reach for and attempt to eat. Instead of introducing purees or foods you feed your baby with a spoon, you let your baby lead the way with finger foods from the beginning. You present soft, bite-sized pieces of food to your baby in his or her high chair tray, and they go for it! Proponents of baby-led weaning argue that it is more natural for babies to eat this way, and they are less likely to overeat. They feel that spoon-feeding leads to more cajoling and force feeding. Do you remember "here comes the airplane"?

The baby-led weaning movement teaches many beneficial principles. I agree that you should allow your baby to start self-feeding as soon as they are able and willing to do it. When they start reaching for their own food, they are more likely to eat when hungry and stop when satisfied. They are also able to explore the variety of flavors and textures of foods themselves. It is beneficial for motor development and the development of proper chewing. However, most babies are not able to self-feed until after nine months of age, which means you may miss out on some opportunities to introduce those stronger flavors that you would like them to become familiar with if your baby seems ready for solids before that age. You must still be deliberate about which foods you wish to expose your baby to. Remember that as the parent you are in charge of what and when, and your baby decides if and how much. Because this is such a critical time in their development of food preference, it is worth putting thought and effort into introducing certain health-promoting foods. Avoid processed foods that are high in sugar, salt, and added fats, and stick to whole natural foods. Also, always supervise your baby. Make sure that they are sitting upright in a high chair, and avoid choking hazards.

Foods to Avoid

Some foods are best avoided during the first year of life either because they are dangerous or because they are not health-promoting. This includes cow's milk, honey, seafood, shellfish, processed meats, processed foods, and juice. I will briefly explain why each of these is not recommended in children under one year of age.

Cow's milk. Cow's milk can cause lots of trouble for little tummies and should not be introduced for children younger than one year of age. Apart from being naturally low in iron, it can cause microscopic bleeding in the gut of infants and can also decrease the absorption of iron, increasing the likelihood of anemia in babies and toddlers.

Honey. Honey can contain spores, which can cause botulism in babies. Adults are usually unaffected by the small amount that can be present in honey, but babies are more susceptible. Botulism causes constipation, weakness, and, ultimately, difficulty breathing in or even death. Babies under the age of one should never consume honey.

Seafood and shellfish. Seafood can contain mercury and other heavy metals and toxins. If you are going to introduce fish to your baby, keep it to once per week and select fish that are low in contaminants. Smaller, bottom-feeding fish like sardines and anchovies are less likely to have high levels of heavy metals, and they are also richer in omega-3 DHA/EPA as they are the fish that are directly eating the algae that produce the omega-3.

Processed meats. Declared a known carcinogen by the World Health Organization, processed meats such as bacon, hot dogs, and deli meats are associated with colon cancer. They are also very high in salt, which is not health-promoting for babies.

Processed foods. Not only are processed foods such as crackers, cookies, candy, and chips low in fiber and antioxidants, they are usually high in fat, salt, and sugar. This introduces the habit of hyper-palatable foods to babies. Hyper-palatable foods are foods that are specially engineered to have added sugar, salt, and fat to increase our desire for them. Eating these foods accustoms our mouths and brains to expect especially pleasing flavors and makes it difficult to stop eating. It can make whole natural foods seem boring and bland in comparison. Keep your baby's diet free of added sugar, salt, and fried foods for as long as possible.

Juice. In the past, juice was recommended as a first food for babies. However, juice is essentially sugar water. The body responds differently to juice than it would to whole fruit because juice is missing fiber and other nutrients that blunt the sharp spike in sugar and insulin. Juice is very sweet and gets babies accustomed to sugary foods. Instead of juice, give babies fruit. It is much healthier because it includes fiber, and most babies love it!

No-No Foods for Baby

Some foods are notorious choking hazards and should be avoided. This includes hard vegetables or fruit, popcorn, and nuts and seeds in their whole form, hot dogs, and whole grapes because they are the perfect size and shape to occlude the windpipe. Babies at this age do tend to occasionally overshoot, put too much into their mouths, and gag and cough. This is actually a protective mechanism that helps the body avoid choking. Most of the time they quickly recover and spit out the food, but always supervise your baby when they are eating. Learn some basic maneuvers such as the finger sweep (if you can see the food) and back blows that you can implement if your child is unable to breathe. See Rescue Maneuvers for a Choking Baby on page 137 for detailed information.

Safe Baby-Feeding Tips

- Always have your child sitting upright in a high chair.

- Always supervise and interact with your baby.

- Offer soft foods until your baby is ready to chew foods with harder texture.

- Cut finger food into bite-sized pieces.

- Avoid choking hazards such as popcorn, nuts, hard veggies, hot dogs, and whole grapes.

Intuitive Eating Practices for Early Eaters

Once your baby starts eating solids, there's a little more to think about and keep track of, but the general concepts stay the same. First, let's review the division of responsibilities. You, the parent, decide what and when your child will eat. Your baby is in charge of if and how much. Whether you are feeding via a bottle, giving solids with a spoon, or allowing your baby to self-feed, respect your child's satiety signals.

When you start feeding your baby solid foods, things have the potential to get more emotional. Some days your baby won't want food and may throw everything on the floor. Other days you may feel like he or she is a ravenous little beast. Also, it may seem like your baby likes a food one day and not the next. This is all normal! Above all, have fun and be relaxed. Just as with breastfeeding and bottle-feeding your baby, you will find a rhythm that works for you. However, remember that learning to accept new foods is all about exploration. Allow your baby to truly explore foods by touching, smelling, and playing with their food. It is very normal for them to put something in their mouths and spit it right back out. It may take between eight to fifteen exposures to a food before a child accepts it. Allowing them this freedom of exploration and trial and error will help your baby develop into a happy and confident eater.

Babies Love Water

When your baby is between six and nine months of age, introduce a sippy cup or a cup with a straw for drinking water. This will get them familiar with drinking from a cup and consuming water. Offer the cup at meals. Before six months of age, do not give your baby water because it can dilute their blood and cause low sodium levels, which is very dangerous.

Babies between six and twelve months generally become hungry every three hours or so. Each child has hunger signals that you will be attuned to over time. However, you may not get it perfectly right every single time, and that's okay. In general, you will find a schedule that mostly matches your baby's hunger signals. If you are a bit too early, they may eat less than usual. If they show indications of hunger earlier than usual, you may have to adjust the schedule and feed earlier than planned. Remember, intuitive eating is about flexibility and adaptability. Also, realize that as your child gets older and you get busier, you may miss a cue every once in a while. Life happens. The worst thing that can happen is you get a cranky baby until you offer them food. Hunger comes in waves, so you have time to acknowledge and respond. Hunger is not an emergency, and this is not a reason to overfeed your baby. Neither should you overfeed in order to prevent hunger later.

To support intuitive eating in your little eaters, offer foods at mealtimes and snack times. As always, make sure that they are sitting, and the environment is pleasant and unrushed. Offer only one or two foods at a time to avoid overwhelming your baby. Then, let your baby take the wheel. If your baby seems uninterested or disgusted, don't despair. Resist the temptation to encourage your child to eat more or try to force food into their mouths. Once they are done, clean up and move on to the next activity.

Continue to offer a variety of health-promoting foods, including choices that may have been previously rejected. Remember, it can take more than fifteen exposures to a food before a child accepts it! The key is consistency and persistence. Children will develop a taste for foods that they are repeatedly exposed to.

Habits to Support Intuitive Eating

1. Always seat your child at a table or high chair with tray.

2. Minimize distractions such as television and phone. Keep music low and calm.

3. Create a pleasant environment.

4. Sit down at the table with your child and enjoy your food too.

5. Allow your baby to truly explore their food by touching, smelling, and even playing with their food.

6. Never force or coerce a child into eating more. When they are done, respect that choice!

7. Consistency and persistence are essential to helping your child acquire the flavor of foods.

Sign Language

Babies can start to learn and use baby sign language sooner than they can talk, and it can be a very useful tool in communication. I used sign language with both of my sons, and it was a lifesaver. The most helpful basic signs to begin with are "eat," "more," "milk," and "all done." You can start making these signs when your baby is around six months old, and wait for your baby to start using them. Some babies will start using them as early as nine months of age, but others may not make their first sign until they are over one year. It's quite amazing being able to communicate with your little one and a great way for them to tell you that they are hungry or full. For recommended resources, visit the resources section at the end of the book.

Key Points

- Don't be afraid to offer a variety of green vegetables and beans, fruits, and nut and seed butters.

- It's okay to get messy! Starting your baby on solids is an adventure. Have fun and don't stress about the mess. Let your baby play and enjoy the colors, textures, and flavors of foods!

- Be patient and persistent. If your baby doesn't like a new food immediately, it's okay! It's very tempting to beg or plead with your baby to eat. Resist the temptation and be sensitive to your baby's hunger and satiety cues. Keep offering that option at other meals.

- Transition to finger foods and allow your baby to self-feed as soon as they show signs of readiness. When babies are able to feed themselves, this allows them to be even more connected to their hunger and satiety signals.

- Begin to establish a routine for meals and snacks but remain sensitive to early hunger and satiety cues.

- Avoid introducing juice, processed foods, and hyper-palatable foods to your baby.

Chapter 13

The Toddler Years:
1 Year through 3 Years

The toddler years are incredible. Suddenly you live with a walking, talking little boss. Toddlers are curious, emotional, expressive, and often hilarious. They are also vocal (and sometimes very dramatic) about their preferences, which seem to change every hour.

Once your little one becomes mobile, the world takes on a whole new allure. The job of a toddler is to explore and play all day long. It can be an exhausting but fun time for parents. Parents of toddlers often come to me in frustration and worry that their child just doesn't sit down and eat. This is common, and it is NORMAL. Toddlers are the ultimate intuitive eaters. They only dare pull themselves away from the most important task of their day if it is very pressing. Toddlers are the CEOs of play, and they take their job very seriously! When they finally do sit down to eat, they eat until they are no longer hungry so they can get back to work, I mean, play. Some days they eat like birds, and some days they eat a ton! As long as they are growing and following their growth curves and development, there is no worry.

Toddlerhood is also a time when many previously "good eaters" that seemed to enjoy a variety of foods start to reject foods. This is also expected.

Especially if they are not very hungry, some kids will see a food and immediately reject it. Your toddler's tummy is only the size of his or her fist. Your task during this stage of development is to be patient, be persistent, and remain confident.

After one year of age, toddlers progress very quickly from walking to running and climbing on everything. Although they do continue to grow and stretch out, the rate of growth slows a bit. Also, many toddlers will often maintain a toddler tummy, which is accentuated by a prominent curve of their lower spine. Although this is typical at this age, some parents worry that their child appears bloated or too chubby around their abdomen.

How to Feed Your Toddler

Transitioning Off the Bottle

After your baby's first birthday, wean off the bottle over one month so that they are bottle-free by thirteen months of age. Keeping your child on a bottle longer than a year increases the risk of cavities and can interfere with the healthy development of the mouth and teeth. By twelve months, babies are taking three to four bottles per day. Start with the bottle that your child is least attached to and replace it with a cup on the first week, then the next easiest one the second week. The third and fourth are usually nap and nighttime bottles. By the end of the month, the baby should be off the bottle completely and taking their milk via a cup. At this point, eliminate all the bottles in the house!

After children are weaned off the bottle, water should become their primary beverage and the *only* thing they drink between meals. You will be offering your child three meals per day in addition to snacks (more on this in the next section). If you choose to give a milk alternative, I recommend a calcium-fortified, *unsweetened* plant-based milk such as soy, coconut, oat, or hemp. There are many to choose from and some are easily made at home. Offer this beverage during meals instead of sipping between meals. Unless you are told differently by your pediatrician, keep the intake of the milk alternative to 16 oz or less per day. Your toddler should now be getting the vast majority of their calories and nutrition from solid food!

Mothers who continue nursing beyond one year of age can continue to breastfeed on demand, but I still do recommend eliminating bottles. Pumped breast milk can be given in a cup at meals if mothers are not directly breastfeeding. After one year of age, I recommend offering solid food before breastfeeding at meals. Some babies are still nursing frequently, and others may have slowed down to just a few times per day.

Night Nursing and Cavities

Once children start eating solid foods, they develop an increased risk of cavities. This can be worsened by frequent nursing at night. The natural sugars in breast milk can augment bacterial processes in the mouth when milk pools there overnight. To avoid an increased risk of cavities, take care to brush your child's teeth twice daily, especially before bed. Take your child to see a dentist after they turn one, and if they start developing cavities and they are frequently nursing at night, it may be a reason to wean from night feeds.

Intuitive Eating for Toddlers

Continue to offer your growing toddler a variety of vegetables, whole grains, beans, and nut and seed butters. Offer these foods within three meals per day as well as during a couple of snacks as needed. Most of the time, your child will be eating what you are eating. Continue to foster healthy eating habits like sitting for meals. This is especially important for toddlers who might become "drive-by" eaters if there is no structure or routine to their meals and eating.

Establish a regular routine for meals and snacks and keep in mind that toddlers may become hungry every two to four hours. Keep a general structure but continue to be flexible and sensitive in responding to hunger cues.

Toddlers who aren't yet using words can continue to use sign language to express their needs and desires; however, most children will start using specific words for their needs by eighteen months. Because toddlers are very active and have a high interest in play and exploring their environment, they may actually ignore or miss their initial hunger signals. This can result in meltdowns and temper tantrums. If this is typical for your toddler, you may have to pay attention and catch them earlier in their hunger wave.

At this age, you can also start using language about hunger and satiety. You can refer to hunger as having an "empty tummy" and satiety as a "full tummy." This is another way to teach children to tune into their bodies.

The biggest mistake that parents make at this point is to start the habit of bribing, cajoling, and bargaining with their child. Parents mean well when they encourage their toddlers to eat just another bite or two or force them to eat their vegetables. I think part of the reason is that at this age children naturally slow down in their weight gain. As they become more active they may also look leaner. As their rate of growth slows, they may have a reduced appetite at times, and it may seem like they don't eat very much, which can provoke anxiety for parents. Parents start to worry that their child is not gaining enough weight, and they may get comments from other family members. They start chasing their child around with food and giving them processed foods or "kid-friendly" foods such as chicken nuggets and grilled cheese sandwiches because "that's all they will eat."

At this stage of development, it is entirely normal for toddlers to have a food jag in their diet and suddenly refuse a food that they previously liked. A food jag is when a child suddenly refuses to eat most foods and prefers to eat only one or a small number of foods for several days in a row. This can be incredibly distressing for parents. Take a deep breath, sit back, and trust your child's intuition. Your job is to offer healthy and regular meals and snacks, and your child's job is to decide if and how much. If they are not hungry and don't eat, don't panic! Just put it away and offer it again at the next meal or snack time.

Speaking of snacks, this is also around the time that snacks become a different category of food, consisting of Goldfish crackers, graham crackers, Cheerios, and "fruit" snacks (that aren't actually made of fruit). But the majority of these snack foods are processed! Snack food doesn't have to be a special category of food! It can be the same food you eat at mealtimes! Fruits, vegetables, whole grains, beans, and nut and seed butters.

Terrific Toddler Snacks

- Fresh fruit (sliced apples, bananas, berries, mandarin orange slices, cut melons)

- Fresh vegetables (cucumber slices, sliced zucchini, bell pepper strips, cauliflower, carrots)

- Freeze-dried fruits

- Cooked whole beans (rinsed chickpeas and kidney beans are perfect!)

- Apple slices with unsweetened peanut butter

- Hummus with raw veggies (see hummus recipe on page 165)

- Whole grain tortilla chips with bean dip

- Plant-based yogurt (soy, almond, and coconut are some examples) with granola

- Rice cakes topped with mashed avocado (see recipe on page 153)

- Whole grain toast topped with mashed fruit

- Green smoothies (see recipes on pages 119 and 120)

- Leftovers from lunch or dinner!

Just like your early eater, toddlers will require lots of persistence and consistency to encourage their preference for a variety of whole plant foods. Even if they reject a specific food over and over, continue to offer it and then step away.

Special Considerations

Overdependence on Breast Milk

Breast milk is sweet, moderate in fat content, and low in protein, and it has around twenty calories per ounce. Some toddlers nurse so frequently or consume so much breast milk that they barely eat solids and start losing weight or having difficulty with normal weight gain. Others may overconsume breast milk and they may miss out on the nutrients in foods as well as the experience of trying new foods and flavors early on. As previously mentioned, breast milk is naturally low in iron, which is a mineral that babies need after six months of age. Mothers should continue to breastfeed as long as it feels right for them. However, if your child is over eighteen months old, not eating solids well, and is either losing weight or not gaining weight, I recommend that you drop the number of nursing episodes per day to see if this improves their appetite.

Juice

Juice is not a necessary part of a child's diet, and there is no reason to introduce it at this age deliberately. For more selective children or children with smaller appetites, juice may abate their hunger and displace more nutritious foods. For other children, liquid calories bypass their satiety signals, and they can end up overconsuming calories. Juice can also cause osmotic or "toddler's" diarrhea. Osmotic diarrhea occurs when undigested sugars enter the colon and draw water with them, leading to several watery stools per day. Because this type of diarrhea can commonly arise with excess juice consumption in little ones, it is also known as toddler's diarrhea. Ironically, in some children the opposite can happen. Pectin is a type of fiber that can cause stools to loosen or firm up. You may be familiar with it being used to make jelly. Apple juice, because of its high pectin content, can actually cause constipation in some children. In addition, children become adapted to the very sweet flavor of juice and may reject water because it starts to taste relatively plain. Finally, it can cause tooth decay, especially if it is sipped throughout the day or right before bed. Avoid deliberately introducing juice into the diet of your baby or toddler or including it as a regular part of their diet. They will have access and exposure to it soon enough in the coming years.

Too Many Vegetables?

There can be such a thing as a child eating too many vegetables at this age. Although it doesn't happen often, occasionally a child can love vegetables and fruit so much they do not eat much else. These foods are very nutritious and contain loads of vitamins and antioxidants, but they are also very low in calories and high in fiber. Consequently, little tummies can fill up before taking in sufficient calories for growth. This is particularly true of raw vegetables. If this is the case for your toddler, start to shift the foods that you offer so that they are getting more beans, nut and seed butters, and whole grains, which are denser in calories.

Recipes for the Toddler Years

Fruity Breakfast Toast

Delicious, nutritious, and fun to eat!

Serves: 1 to 2

2 slices whole grain or whole wheat bread (no added oil, dairy, or egg)

2 to 4 tablespoons unsweetened peanut butter, nut butter, or seed butter (can also use a plant-based yogurt, such as soy, coconut, or almond yogurt)

½ cup diced fruit of your choice (bananas, strawberries, blueberries, raspberries)

1. Toast the bread.

2. Spread a thin layer of nut butter on each piece of toast then top with fruit.

3. Cut into bite-sized squares and serve.

Chickpea Salad

A fiber-full take on tuna sandwiches that is sure to please!

Serves: 4

1 (15-ounce) can chickpeas, drained and rinsed

¼ cup vegan mayonnaise (such as Just Mayo or Vegenaise)

2 teaspoons seaweed flakes (optional)

½ teaspoon onion powder

½ teaspoon dried dill

2 tablespoon bread and butter pickles, chopped

whole grain bread, whole wheat tortillas, or salad, to serve

a parent's guide to intuitive eating

1. Roughly mash the chickpeas in a bowl with a fork. Add the vegan mayo, spices, and bread and butter pickles, and mix well.

2. Spread on slices of whole grain bread, wrap in a whole wheat tortilla, or serve over a salad. Delicious with lettuce and tomatoes!

The Easiest Black Bean Chili Ever

I learned this recipe as a Food for Life instructor. Anybody can prepare this simple recipe and it is amazingly tasty!

Serves: 4

2 (15-ounce) cans black beans (low sodium if possible), undrained

1 (16-ounce) jar mild salsa

8 ounces frozen sweet corn, thawed

cooked brown rice, to serve

guacamole and chopped cilantro, to top (optional)

Mix the black beans, salsa, and corn together in a saucepan and gently warm over medium heat for 15 minutes. Serve over fresh brown rice and top with guacamole and cilantro, if using.

Rice Cakes with Mashed Avocado

It's like avocado toast, only crunchier and incredibly simple. Your toddler will love it!

Serves: 1 to 2

¼ cup mashed avocado or guacamole

2 brown rice cakes

Spread the avocado on the rice cakes and enjoy!

Key Points

- Wean your child off the bottle at one year of age. Water should be a child's main beverage and what they drink between meals.

- Continue to offer three meals per day, plus snacks as needed.

- Continue to emphasize vegetables, fruits, whole grains, beans, and nut and seed butters.

- Be persistent and consistent; keep your cool.

- Avoid processed foods, "kid-friendly" and "snack" foods, as well as juice and other sweet beverages.

- Avoid drinking milk between meals, before bedtime, or throughout the night as it increases the risk of cavities.

Chapter 14

Preschool and the Early School Years: 4 Years through 10 Years

Your preschooler is now fully conversational and learning new skills at the speed of light. Your child can play imaginatively, play cooperatively with other children, and sing a song. Once your child is four or five, they will likely start going to school, playgroups, or other public settings. Going to school is exciting and comes with a different set of challenges. Regular exposure to a world of food outside of the home can be both thrilling and daunting. Learning to navigate the school years and find your rhythm and routine may take some practice, but once you get it, it'll be a piece of cake (figuratively for you and literally for your child).

Over the next few years, your child will continue to grow and stretch, eventually losing that toddler's tummy and appearing leaner. This continues until puberty begins. Some girls will start to have early puberty signs around age nine. Once the hormones start changing, girls will begin to store fat around the thighs, hips, and breasts, which is a very normal part of human development.

Loosening the Reins

Once your child is out in the world, you lose some of the control over what they are offered. At this stage, start allowing some freedom of choice along with gentle and trusting guidance. You must continue to trust your child and not panic when they make food choices that you are uncomfortable with. However, don't forget that you are still the gatekeeper in the home.

After you have instilled the principles of intuitive eating in your household and your child goes out into the world, it will be time to loosen the reins. You will still be there to guide and gently influence, but you must allow your child the freedom to explore. If you give them trust, they will learn to trust themselves. Continue to keep your home a health-promoting, safe place, and your child will continue to learn and use the skills of intuitive eating even when they are not at home.

Introducing Play Foods

I love the term "play foods," coined by Evelyn Tribole and Elyse Resch in the book, *Intuitive Eating*. Play foods are foods that are usually processed and may not be very health-promoting, yet we choose to eat them because they are delicious or culturally significant, and they bring us pleasure. These foods may not be packed with antioxidants or fiber, but they do have value in our lives. A perfect example of play food is birthday cake. We don't eat birthday cake every day, but when we do it is a fun and celebratory experience, and it brings us joy. Although infants and toddlers may not be exposed to these foods, once children are old enough, they start to experience these foods and may come to like them. It is critical that once children discover these foods and desire them, they be allowed to have some. You can start to talk to your children about why we like these foods, why it may not be beneficial to make them the central part of our diet, and how consuming them in excess or with frequency can make us feel physically and emotionally. Help them tune into their bodies so they can use this feedback to make eating decisions that are appropriate for them.

Play Food Drawer

I was inspired by emotional eating expert Josie Spinardi, author of *How to Have Your Cake and Skinny Jeans Too*, to develop the concept of a play food "drawer." The idea is to give your child their own drawer or cabinet (preferably in the kitchen or pantry) to keep a small stash of his or her preferred "play food." It is a great way to avoid restriction and allow your child a little more freedom and choice. When I first started applying the principles of intuitive eating to my children, I let go of the tight reins of control and made play food drawers for everyone in the household—even me. Actually, I think I benefitted the most. If you don't already know what your child's favorite play foods are, ask them and purchase a small amount once a week or month to place in their special area. They then have the freedom to choose when to eat it. I guide my children to avoid eating these foods right before a meal or after they brush their teeth at night; otherwise, I don't comment or interfere. This may seem like a scary, wild thing to do. Believe me, I was petrified when I began using this method at home, but it had amazing results. If your child is accustomed to being restricted, they may visit this drawer often in the beginning, but over time, especially if you do not become critical or disapproving of their choice to eat these foods, the frequency will decrease. My younger son has some candy in his drawer that's more than a year old. Now everybody in the house has their designated area where they know their special treats will be safe and they will not be judged for eating these items.

How to Feed Your School-Age Child

At this age, especially if you have already established good eating habits, you will continue to offer a variety of whole plant foods. However, you will have to make some choices about foods outside of the home.

School Lunch

Daycares and preschools that receive federal subsidies for their food program are required to comply with federal guidelines. Current guidelines include a minimum amount of dairy, fruits, vegetables, specific requirements for "protein," and even legumes in the menu each week. While they've improved significantly over time, school lunches still often contain processed meats and a fair amount of dairy and cheese. If you are allowed to bring your own food, you may be required by the school to ensure that your child's lunch box contains components that comply with the guidelines for the macronutrients.

The option of eating a school lunch can have advantages. It can be cost-effective (especially if you qualify for free lunch), convenient, and perhaps more desirable to some children who want to do what all the other kids do. The disadvantages include the amount of processed meats, including the quantity of deli meats, hot dogs, sausages, and pepperoni, and the dairy present in school lunches.

Another disadvantage of the school lunch is that some children dislike it because it is different from what they eat at home, and they may not eat much.

How you choose to approach school lunch for your child is up to you. Some families elect to have their child always eat school lunch, and others choose to send their child to school with a sack lunch. Of course, you could also choose a combination. You can review the menu with your child, and they can select some meals they like at school and take their sack lunch on other days.

Packing your child's lunch does not have to be overwhelming once you get the hang of it. Make sure to include fruits, veggies, beans, whole grains, and a little bit of play food too. Below are some lunch box ideas.

Main dishes:

- Hummus wraps or sandwiches with veggies such as cucumber, tomatoes, red bell pepper, shredded carrots, and pickles (see page 165)

- Avocado whole grain bagel sandwiches with tomato and lettuce

- Chickpea salad sandwiches (see page 152)

- Whole fruit such as apples, bananas, grapes, kiwis, or cherries

- Raw, cut-up veggies such as broccoli, cauliflower, carrots, celery, and red bell pepper strips with hummus or white bean dip

- Homemade veggie sushi

- Sunflower seed butter and jelly sandwiches on whole grain or whole wheat bread

- Fruit roll-ups: whole grain tortilla with seed butter, jelly, and bananas, strawberries, or fruit of your choice (see page 165)

- Bean burritos and corn chips with salsa

- Falafel in pita bread sandwiches

- Roasted veggies with pasta

- Minestrone soup with whole grain bread

Side items:

- Applesauce

- Pretzels, whole grain chips, or crispy chickpeas

- Olives

- Granola bars

- Whole grain muffin bites

Parties and Special Events

The challenge doesn't end with school lunches. School has become a place of seemingly constant celebration. For the average size class, there seems to be at least one birthday per week and holiday celebrations never end. Some teachers still reward with candy and edible treats. Don't forget the numerous bake sales, fundraisers, and other school celebrations involving lots of processed foods, candy, and sweets. The first time your child comes home looking like a very jolly Smurf after eating a blue cupcake, take a deep breath, and don't panic.

There are several ways you can approach these treat foods. The first is just to allow things to be as they are. Yes, that is a valid choice, and although it may raise your blood pressure, it is unlikely to harm your child in any permanent way. Continue to keep your home as health-promoting as possible and help your child learn the difference between health-promoting foods and those that are not quite as health-promoting. You can also teach your children how to tune into their bodies to assess how certain processed foods make them feel. However, if you make this choice, do not judge, guilt, or shame your child if they choose to eat these foods. Saying phrases such as, "You've had enough junk food," "That food is fattening," or "That food is bad for you," or even giving a simple judging look can interfere with your child's ability to self-regulate their intake. Doing so can cause problems in the future.

Another option is to bring a stash of shelf-stable (nut-free if your school requires it), plant-based alternatives that the teacher can keep in her classroom to give your child when there is a celebration. That way, your child gets a "treat," one that you have provided with ingredients that you are comfortable with. This is what I did when my children were younger. Once they got into the junior high stage, I stopped doing it and just let them make their own choices at school. It took a lot to let go, but it felt right for us.

Another choice some parents make is to request that their child not participate at all. This might be exceedingly difficult. Some children have to do this because of extreme food allergies. Children really look forward to these celebrations, and whether it is right or wrong to have so many, not being allowed to participate at all could lead to a disordered relationship with food. They may feel deprived and isolated and want to have that food even more. You have to explore what is right for you and your family, and this choice may evolve over time.

Navigating the school years when you deeply desire your child to eat a health-promoting diet is not easy but is a great learning opportunity for both you and your children. Remember that in general, kids do great, and some processed foods here and there are not going to cause long-term damage. As children are given more freedom and space to decide and as they learn more about health-promoting foods and how processed foods make them feel, they will usually gravitate toward eating more whole plant foods when they are allowed to make their own decisions.

Including Children in Meal Planning and Cooking

This is the perfect age to include your child in the meal planning, shopping, and preparation of food. It serves several purposes. It allows them to gain more knowledge about health-promoting foods, it gives them choice, and it starts to teach them the invaluable skill of meal planning and preparation. You don't have to involve your kids in every little detail, but the more you include them, the more excited they will be to eat the foods you prepare together. As I am meal planning each week, I ask my family if they have any specific requests for the week. Sometimes they do, and sometimes they don't. Take your child to the grocery store with you, and allow them to choose the produce on the shopping list or pick a fruit or vegetable they would like to eat that week. In the kitchen, involve your child by letting them wash produce, measure ingredients, stir, and mix. Once they are old enough, they can do some supervised chopping. Around the age of ten, they can start to learn some easy recipes that they can help make and prepare on their own with supervision. These are useful life skills, but it also increases the chance that your child will continue to eat healthfully once they leave your home.

Special Considerations

Food Battles

I remember many evenings when I spent an hour or two preparing a beautiful and delicious meal, only to be met with looks of disgust, turned-up noses, and grumpy dispositions. In turn, I became defensive and irritable, insisting that my children eat the food I made. Tears and emotional drama ensued. This would happen again the next night...and the next. I know exactly what it feels like to be stuck in the cycle of food wars. Thankfully, I learned how to avoid those battles altogether. Now dinner feels fun and relaxed, and there are (rarely) any tears.

Since my oldest son started eating solids, he was interested in and accepting of most foods. He would try almost anything and was not hesitant or anxious about new foods. I remember him delightfully tasting spicy salsa repeatedly when he was a mere fifteen months old.

However, my second son is a different story. When I would present a meal that was unfamiliar or unexpected, he would immediately pout, and often cry and refuse to eat. Back then, this would make me anxious, so I would beg and plead, which often led to more tears. He eventually would eat it (and actually like it), but I felt like I had just run a marathon by the end of dinner. Even worse, my older son decided that he would start complaining about the food too! I guess he never knew he had that option before. Then I had two grumpy kids staring at the dinner that I had spent time and energy preparing for them! How could they?! It took me a while to learn, but I finally developed a strategy that lowered the stress and battles at our table.

How to Avoid Food Battles

Prepare your child. Children who are anxious about new things need time to mentally prepare for new food encounters. Let your child know well ahead of time prior to offering an unfamiliar meal or cuisine. Validate your child's emotions by saying something like, "I know it may make you feel nervous and it's probably not what you prefer to eat, and that's okay."

Make it easier. Put something that you know they like with the rest of the food, especially if you are introducing something new. This helps relieve some of the stress your child might feel.

Don't force it. Never force a child to eat. I think the most stressful part of food battles for a child is feeling pressured to eat when they are not hungry or when they are incredibly anxious.

Don't beg or plead. This is similar to forcing. It is stressful for you, and it is often unsuccessful. Keep your calm, and stay on your plan.

Store it. Save your child's food for later if they choose not to eat. If there are times that my child isn't hungry or simply chooses not to eat dinner, I will save it and 99 percent of the time, he will come back and eat it before bed when his appetite is finally strong enough to outweigh his resistance to the food.

Make it a game or a challenge. Another technique that I have employed with my children is to create a food challenge, such as eating vegetables or trying new foods. Each person in the family gets points (or some sort of nonfood reward) for eating more vegetables or for being brave and trying new foods. Turning it into a game often takes out the anxiety for many children, especially when they see other family members trying their best.

Chill out. Take lots of deep breaths, relax, and do not take it personally. This one is probably the hardest. Staying calm can be hard on days when you are tired and feel emotionally drained and unappreciated. Who wants to present the most beautiful casserole to a table of pouting faces? You won't be perfect at this, but with practice, you will get better at these skills and it will no longer be the battle it used to be. One day you'll look up and realize that you have created an atmosphere of fun and harmony at the table!

Reality Check: Are You a Short-Order Cook?

You may wonder why you can't just make everyone their favorite meal or food to keep the peace. Well, the truth is you can if you really want to. Remember, you are the boss! However, I don't recommend it. First of all, it is stressful and time consuming to cook and prepare separate meals for everyone. It's hard enough finding the time to prepare *one* nutritious meal! Second, many children's preferred food to eat may not be health-promoting. Third, offering the same food over and over without variety will cause them to stay stuck in a restricted pattern. In general, I recommend keeping the main family meal the same for everyone. For most households in the United States, this will be dinner. For their breakfast or lunch box, you may allow your children a little more choice if you have the time and ability.

There are also ways to include more choice and flexibility at dinner to allow for individual taste preferences. Make meals that allow for freedom of choice, such as a salad, taco, or baked potato bar, or make-your-own pizza where children can pick their own toppings. These types of meals allow children to choose their own toppings and accommodates all taste preferences. Avoid creating completely separate meals for the children. If mom and dad are having tacos for dinner, the kids shouldn't be offered mac and cheese. Not every meal that you make is going to be your child's favorite meal, and that is okay. Make meals delicious and enjoyable, but don't expect them to please everyone perfectly.

Recipes for Preschool and the Early School Years

Fruity Roll-Ups

This is my youngest son's favorite breakfast. Quick and easy to make and tastes like a treat!

Serves: 1

1 whole wheat, whole grain, or gluten-free tortilla or wrap

2 tablespoons peanut butter or other nut butter (can also use plant-based yogurt or applesauce)

½ cup diced fruit of your choice (bananas and strawberries work very well)

Spread the nut butter or plant-based yogurt on the tortilla. Top with the diced fruit. Roll up and enjoy!

Hummus and Veggie Wraps

These wraps are so simple and scrumptious! Get creative with the veggies. Sliced red and yellow bell peppers look beautiful in this wrap. Assembled they will last three days in the fridge. This makes a great lunch box item.

Serves: 4 to 6

2 (15-ounce) cans chickpeas, drained and rinsed

2 tablespoons roasted sunflower seeds (for a yummy nutty flavor!)

2 tablespoons lemon juice

2 tablespoons soy sauce (or tamari)

1 teaspoon garlic powder

½ teaspoon cumin

½ teaspoon smoked paprika

¼ cup water

whole wheat or whole grain tortillas or wraps

shredded carrots

baby spinach

1. Add the chickpeas, sunflower seeds, lemon juice, soy sauce or tamari, garlic powder, cumin, smoked paprika, and water to a blender and blend until smooth.

2. Spread the hummus on a tortilla and then line with a layer of shredded carrots followed by a layer of spinach.

3. Roll up and enjoy! You can also slice into pretty pinwheels.

Pita Pizzas

Kids get really excited about pizza. These can be baked in the oven or eaten plain like a pita pocket. Either way, kids will enjoy creating their own personal healthy pizza. Get creative with toppings and include other vegetables, beans, and herbs.

Serves: 6

1 cup pasta sauce

6 whole grain pita breads

1 cup thinly sliced carrot rounds

1 cup sliced black olives

1 cup sliced mushrooms

1. Spread 2 tablespoons of sauce on a piece of pita. Top with the carrots, olives, and mushrooms.

2. You can then either fold up and eat, or bake for 10 minutes in an oven that has been preheated to 350°F.

Happy Rancher Dip

Kids love to dip! This recipe is inspired by ranch dressing, which is beloved by children. However, this version is loaded with fiber. The cashews give it an irresistible creamy texture that keeps kids coming back for more. This also works great as a dressing when thinned with extra water.

Serves: 6

½ cup unsweetened nondairy milk (such as soy)

1 cup raw cashews (soaked for at least 4 hours)

½ cup cannellini beans

½ teaspoon garlic powder

½ teaspoon onion powder

2 green onions

½ teaspoon sea salt

¼ cup chopped fresh parsley

raw vegetables, to serve

1. Blend together all the ingredients except the parsley in a blender until very smooth. Add the parsley and pulse to desired consistency.

2. Serve with raw veggies such as carrots, broccoli, cauliflower, bell pepper slices, and sliced zucchini.

Key Points

- Start to allow your child more freedom in food choices outside of the home at school, parties, and restaurants.

- Consider integrating a play food drawer for your child at home.

- Involve your child in menu planning, grocery shopping, and meal preparation.

- Continue to talk to your child about the feeling of hunger, fullness, and other body sensations.

- Pressuring your child to eat leads to stressful food battles. Decrease the stress by sticking to the habits.

- Avoid becoming a short-order cook. Prepare one health-promoting dinner for the family.

Chapter 15

Tweens and Teens:
11 Years through 18 Years

I n my last two years of high school, I had early release. Because I finished at 1 p.m. and was always staying up later than I should, I would skip breakfast AND lunch and, on the way home, stop at a gas station to buy a large bag of Fritos that I would eat while driving home. Looking back, I'm appalled at my own choices, but I honestly didn't know better.

Oh, the teen years! Teenagers are fascinating creatures because they are learning to become their own person, express themselves, and decide for themselves what they want to believe and be part of. However, their frontal lobe is not fully developed, so they do still have trouble with decision-making and understanding the long-term consequences of their actions. I have always been accepting of the possibility that my sons may not choose to eat in this way in the future when they are out on their own. However, I have never let them forget why we make the food choices we do now.

From age eleven onward, children are starting the transition into adolescence and early adulthood. The majority of children have entered puberty, and this surge of hormones causes changes in their physical appearance as well as their social and emotional lives. Girls will develop more fat around their hips, thighs, and breasts. They also have a growth spurt sooner than boys. Boys start to lose body fat and build more lean muscle. Both boys and girls begin to become more interested in their appearance and spending more time with their friends. In this developmental stage, social acceptability becomes even more significant, and children start to worry more about what their friends think. This normal developmental shift can leave some children vulnerable to eating disorders. However, it is also a time when some children may start behaving more like their friends to fit in. Besides wanting to dress like their friends or have the latest phone, some children may start eating like their friends too. This may lead them to experiment with foods and eating in ways that they previously haven't.

Despite all of this growth and striving for independence, tweens and teens are still children and need the guidance and safety of healthy boundaries. Although they may seem perfectly capable of taking care of their own needs and start pulling away from you, continue to model and reinforce those healthy habits and behaviors that you established early that will set them up for a long, healthy life. However, it will require patience, tolerance, and non-judgement.

How to Feed Your Older Child

Your child may now be making even more food choices outside of the home, which means that maintaining a health-promoting home is even more critical. Continue to provide a variety of whole plant foods and do what you can to make these foods as convenient and accessible as possible. Children at this age can put together some of their own meals and snacks but will tend to grab what is fast and easy. Continue to prepare delicious, nutritious meals centered around whole plant foods. Have a regular routine that is flexible and adaptable to life changes in this busy stage. Continue to also include some play foods in the diet during meals or in their play food drawer.

At this stage, children may take a more significant role in menu planning and meal preparation. Some teens may enjoy preparing meals for the family occasionally. This is a great way to continue to reinforce those health-promoting skills that they can take with them to college and beyond.

Easy Access Foods for Your Teen

- Fruit bowl on the countertop (apples, oranges, bananas)

- Cut-up fresh fruit in the fridge (grapes, melons, berries)

- Washed and prepared fresh vegetables (carrots, broccoli and cauliflower florets, red bell pepper strips)

- Hummus and other bean dips

- Whole grain crackers

- Raw unsalted nuts (almonds, cashews, walnuts, pistachios)

- Whole grain muffins

- Homemade granola bars

- Cooked grains (brown rice, quinoa, oatmeal)

- Cooked beans (chickpeas, black beans, kidney beans, pinto beans, edamame)

- Leftovers from lunch and dinner

Intuitive Eating for Tweens and Teens

Discussing Health with Teens

How you broach the topic of food, body, and health can be either helpful or harmful. Studies show that focusing on body size, or weight tends to lead to disordered and unhealthy eating patterns but discussing health and well-being leads to more balanced eating choices. Set the best example you can of being healthy and joyful and, with time, your teen might come along. The more you push, the more resistance you may encounter.

Another Plug for Family Meals

If you haven't already gotten into the habit of family meals (page 111), this is the stage where it is enormously beneficial. It doesn't have to be every day, but even a few nights per week provides many benefits to children and adolescents. Plus, it is a great way to spend time with your rapidly growing child while enjoying a nourishing meal.

Special Considerations

Bringing Food into the Home

Once teens start driving and have some spending money of their own, the world of food opens up even further. You may start seeing the appearance of foods in your home that have not previously been available. Suddenly, soda, chips, cookies, and fast-food items may begin appearing on your counters.

This can be a frustrating time. The way that you approach it will influence how your child continues to make food decisions. Maintaining calm and patience during this stage is critical. However, it is acceptable and beneficial to set a few boundaries. One boundary may be encouraging your child to save their appetite for the family meals that are planned. Another may be asking them to place their play foods out of sight or in the play food drawer, especially if there are younger children or other family members in the house who may have a difficult time seeing play foods every time they walk into the kitchen. Hopefully, you have a good relationship with your teen, and you can be open and communicate about choices that cause you anxiety. Refrain from shaming or guilting your child, and remember that you were a teen once too.

Young Athletes

There's a common concern that eating a predominantly plant-based diet is not adequate for serious athletes (both children and adults). Evidence shows it is not only sufficient but may provide benefits in recovery and performance. However, when it comes to children, special considerations apply. When children become serious competitive athletes, they may be physically active for several hours each day. Naturally, their bodies will require greater calories. However, athletes should continue to obey their appetite, eating when they are hungry and stopping when they are satisfied. If they are burning more calories with their physical activity, they will have to bridge this gap by eating more substantial quantities of food or eating more frequently, following their hunger drives. If your athlete does not enjoy consuming large amounts of food and gets easily satisfied with smaller portions, you may need to concentrate on increasing the calorie density of the food by adding in nuts, seeds, and nut seed butters, beans, and whole grains. You can make some homemade granola bars containing nut butter or a variety of nuts, homemade trail mix with dried fruit and raw nuts, chocolate coconut balls, and other calorie-dense snacks packed with fiber and antioxidants. You can also concentrate calories in smoothies by adding nut butters, beans, and whole grains like oats. Many successful high-profile athletes eat a whole food, plant-based diet and are at the top of their game.

One of the common things that I see happening with competitive athletes at this age is that they get into the habit of eating highly processed convenience foods because it is easy and does not seem to be affecting them negatively. They may be lean, muscular, and feel "fine," so they don't think that it is a problem. However, frequently consuming these processed foods and not emphasizing enough whole plant foods can start to lead to medical problems such as constipation, acne, poor sleep, or mood changes.

Around these teenage years, some children start consuming sports and energy drinks. Children should not consume energy drinks—ever. They can be very dangerous. Often unregulated, they may contain herbal ingredients that can be harmful. Sports drinks are also overemphasized and tend to contain lots of sugar and artificial ingredients. Water is the ultimate beverage for hydration, but if they are practicing for more than two hours or are sweating profusely, they may benefit from a beverage with electrolytes to replace the sodium and potassium lost in sweat. Ensure that your athlete is maintaining adequate hydration before, during, and after practice or games, and realize that if you live in a hot or dry climate, they may need even more than you think. Make sure that they are frequently urinating and the urine is clear to light yellow. For the children who would benefit from an electrolyte replacement beverage, coconut water is an excellent option because it contains electrolytes and usually no additives or artificial dyes, but there are also other products on the market that avoid artificial flavors and colors.

Finally, it is essential to optimize other aspects of your athlete's diet and lifestyle by providing a multivitamin and ensuring adequate sleep and rest. (See Part III for more on optimizing habits.)

Recipes for Tweens and Teens

Overnight Oats

Overnight oats is my very favorite breakfast! I like to store mine in mason jars so that the individual portions are ready to go in the morning. This recipe is easy to adapt with different fruits and nuts that your child enjoys. Delicious cold or warmed!

Serves: 1

½ cup rolled oats

¾ cup unsweetened plant milk (such as soy, almond, or rice milk)

½ teaspoon vanilla extract

1 tablespoon maple syrup (optional)

½ cup chopped fresh or frozen fruit of your choice, such as blueberries, strawberries, pineapple, or mango

2 tablespoons chopped walnuts, almonds, pecans, peanuts, or other nut

1. Combine the oats, milk, vanilla, maple syrup, and fruit in a 12- or 16-ounce mason jar. Top with the nuts.

2. Cover with the lid and refrigerate overnight. Store for 3 to 5 days in the refrigerator.

Easy Black Bean and Rice Burritos

Great for lunch, snack, or dinner, and a flash to whip up. Perfectly filling and nutritious for your growing teen.

Serves: 2

¾ cup cooked brown rice

¾ cup cooked black beans

2 whole wheat or whole grain tortillas

½ cup mashed avocado or guacamole

salsa (optional)

1. Heat up the beans and rice and divide among two tortillas.

2. Top with the avocado and salsa. Roll up and enjoy!

Easy Creamy Tomato Pasta with Broccoli

A weeknight meal that takes less than 30 minutes to prepare and uses only one pot!

Serves: 4 to 6

1 (16-ounce) package whole grain pasta

1 (24-ounce) jar pasta sauce

½ cup raw cashews (soaked for 4 to 12 hours for smoother texture)

½ cup nutritional yeast*

1 pound frozen or fresh vegetables, chopped (frozen broccoli is my favorite!)

1 (15-ounce) can kidney beans, drained

1. Cook the pasta according to package instructions. Set a timer for cooking time minus 7 minutes for frozen veggies (minus 5 minutes for fresh veggies).

2. In the meantime, add the pasta sauce, cashews, and nutritional yeast to a blender. Blend until very smooth.

3. Add the frozen veggies to the boiling water in the last 7 minutes; if using fresh veggies, add in the last 5 minutes. Drain the pasta and veggies and set aside.

4. Heat a pan over low heat and add sauce and beans. Gently warm.

5. Turn off the heat and add the pasta and veggies to the sauce. Mix well. Serve and enjoy!

Nutritional yeast is an inactivated yeast that lends a cheesy flavor to food. It is yellow in color and comes in a powder or flake. It can be found in the bulk section or natural foods section of your grocery store.

Easy Roasted Chickpeas

A high-fiber and high-flavor crispy snack that is super easy to make.

Serves: 6

2 (15-ounce) cans low-sodium chickpeas, drained and rinsed

2 tablespoons taco seasoning

1. Preheat the oven to 350°F.

2. Combine the chickpeas and taco seasoning.

3. Lightly spray a baking sheet with oil. Line the chickpeas on the baking sheet in one layer and place in oven.

4. Roast for 30 minutes, turning halfway through, until golden brown and crunchy.

Key Points

- Respect the independence and choices of your child but continue to set loving boundaries.

- Continue to offer and provide a wide variety of whole plant foods but make them convenient and accessible.

- Continue the habit of family meals, even if it is just a few times per week.

- Discuss food and eating in terms of health and well-being instead of body size or weight.

- Continue to involve your child in menu planning, shopping, and meal preparation.

- Avoid judging, nagging, or shaming your child about their food choices.

Chapter 16

Special Situations That Apply to All Ages

Dessert

I did not grow up eating dessert regularly after a meal and, because of this, it is not something that I regularly offer to my children. However, I know some families that include it after every dinner as a bargaining chip. A few years ago, I encountered a mother of one of my patients who actually felt guilty if she didn't provide several options for dessert at every dinner because eating dessert brought back warm memories from her childhood. I don't think you must or even should offer dessert after every dinner, but it is not harmful to provide it occasionally. If you do offer it regularly, your children may come to expect it and feel disappointed without it. An occasional dessert seems more special. If you *do* offer dessert, resist using it as a bribe for eating vegetables. I also recommend that you pre-portion dessert and offer it with the meal. And remember that dessert doesn't have to be elaborate to be delicious. Even a small piece of chocolate is a sweet way to end a meal.

Eating Out

Eating out is a convenience and a treat. It can serve as a relief to moms and dads who get to skip the cooking and dishes, and it is sometimes a necessity when traveling. However, regularly eating out at restaurants makes it more challenging to stay aligned with health-promoting habits. Food at restaurants is loaded with salt, refined fats, and sugars, and portions are often at least 30 percent larger than they would be at home. Eating out is also more expensive than eating home-cooked meals. While there is no need to eliminate eating out, I recommend that you come up with a plan for how often you and your family will eat out at restaurants. Intuitive eating can be practiced anywhere, including restaurants, and it is a great place to let your children experience the freedom of choosing their own meals and foods.

Children are usually old enough to start choosing their own restaurant meals when they are in the school years. When they are toddlers, you can order for them, and when they are in preschool and too young to read, you can offer them a couple of choices. For toddlers who haven't been exposed to many play foods, continue to order food similar to the health-promoting foods that they are familiar with. Once they are older, they may want to explore a bit more. Some children will be more adventurous when eating out and may want to try foods that they have never tasted before, and others may be more cautious and stick to the old standbys. By now, your child may be interested in having a soft drink or juice at dinner, or perhaps ordering a dessert. It is acceptable to set some boundaries, such as allowing only one or the other or getting a dessert for the entire family to share.

Certain cuisines lend themselves very well to plant-based eating and have a greater offering of vegetables, whole grains, and legumes. These are usually ethnic foods such as Mexican, Chinese, Japanese, and Mediterranean. You don't have to order from the kids' menu for your children. Scan the entire menu for items that can be paired together, such as steamed vegetables and roasted potatoes or a veggie burger patty with a fruit cup, and ask the server if the kitchen is willing to create a meal based on side items.

Most children will likely not finish their entire restaurant meal. Restaurant portions are oversized, and many restaurants are loud and very stimulating so children may be distracted, have a more difficult time focusing, and take longer to eat. Never force them to finish. Instead, be prepared to take their leftovers home to enjoy at another meal.

Be patient, open-minded, and have some flexibility. It will get easier over time as you become an expert at eating out. The good news is that kids are usually satisfied with simple foods. My kids' favorite restaurant meal is beans and rice at the local Mexican restaurant. Ironically, that is also the most common food at home, but when it is accompanied by chips, salsa, and a festive environment, it becomes a treat.

Also be aware that it is not impossible to make health-promoting choices at restaurants, even fast-food establishments. On my Veggie Doctor TV YouTube channel, I have a series of videos entitled "How a Pediatrician Orders at..." in which I show viewers how to order plant-based meals at many popular fast-food chain restaurants.

Easy Health-Promoting Choices at Restaurants

Mexican: refried beans and rice (or pinto beans and rice), veggie burrito, or bean burrito

Japanese: veggie sushi, miso soup, noodles and veggies

Chinese: stir-fried vegetable or tofu with steamed rice

Mediterranean: hummus and pita bread, falafel

American: veggie burger with steamed broccoli and fruit

Steakhouse: baked potato and veggies, plain pasta with marinara sauce and steamed veggies

Intuitive Eating at Restaurants

- Choose meals for toddlers.

- Allow young, school-age kids choice, but help narrow their choices.

- Older kids might know exactly what they want, or they may need help choosing.

- Avoid judging their choice.

- Set some rules. For example, if they order a soft drink, they will not order a dessert, and vice versa.

- Don't forget that restaurant portions are oversized! Don't force your child to finish their meal. Take home a doggy bag!

- Praise your child for being brave and trying something new, but don't be upset if they don't like it.

Road Trips and Vacations

Travel with kids can be so fun and so exhausting! Does anybody else feel that they need a vacation when they return from vacation? Vacation can sometimes feel like a long free-for-all when it comes to eating. Not only is it socially acceptable to eat a considerable amount of highly processed foods, but it is also expected that one will overeat on vacation as usually occurs on cruises and all-inclusive resorts. However, you don't have to promote this mentality for your family. Yes, you can have fun on vacation and experience different foods and tastes, but you can also still emphasize health-promoting foods and intuitive eating during your trip.

One easy thing to do is take convenient health-promoting foods with you. Items that are easy to travel with and bring on an airplane include home-made trail mix, granola bars, fruit, powdered peanut butter, baby carrots, and other cut-up veggies. You can also bring small packets of hummus, peanut butter, and guacamole as long as they fit in your clear quart-sized bag. These foods are great for snacks or to supplement meals on long trips where mealtimes may be unpredictable.

Once you arrive at your destination, there are other things you can do to give yourself more flexibility with food. When I travel with my family, I try to book a room that has a kitchenette or at least a fridge and microwave for the flexibility of preparing at least some of our meals. Many hotels are happy to accommodate this request. For extended family vacations that are one week or longer, we usually rent a condo, and we like to make our own breakfast, pack our lunch, and cook at least half of our dinners. This is a great way to save money, save time, and cut down on the excess calories, salt, and oil that are served at restaurants. We do make it a point to go out a few times and enjoy the local restaurants and cuisine.

If you are traveling by car, you have much more flexibility. We take at least one or two coolers full of our basics, and that makes it much easier to stay on track once we arrive at our destination.

International travel can be a little trickier because you may not be able to bring fresh foods through customs. Depending on your travel destination, you may also be limited as to what you can purchase when you arrive. For these types of trips, it is worth spending time researching your options and planning ahead. There are some ways to get really creative with packaged foods, such as dehydrated soups, granola bars, and freeze-dried foods.

During vacation, be cautious of falling into the free-for-all mentality, and keep modeling and promoting the principles of intuitive eating. Also, be aware that changes in schedule and time zones may throw off digestion and influence hunger signals. Children may eat more or less than usual or at odd times. Continue to follow cues and respect satiety signals.

Although it takes more thought and planning to eat a health-promoting diet during vacation, it is totally doable and worth the effort. You will feel so much better during and AFTER vacation. It is so pleasant to avoid that post-vacation bloat and sluggish feeling of eating too many processed foods. And, really, vacation is mostly about the experience of being somewhere new to explore and with family.

Grandparents and Other Family Members

Grandparents are some of the best people on Earth. In fact, they are so cool that I can't wait to be one! Many children start to spend more time with their grandparents by the time they are toddlers. In my pediatric practice, I see more and more grandparents that are heavily involved in the care of their grandchildren. This provides many benefits for children, parents, and grandparents. Grandparents that help care for their grandchildren may actually live longer!

One of the reasons that grandparents are so wonderful is that they adore their grandchildren and will do almost anything for them. We are lucky at my house because my parents live with us six months out of the year. My kids love being with their grandparents, and they have built special memories with their grandparents that will last forever. However, I have to admit that learning to balance my desires for my kids' nutrition with my parents' choices hasn't always been easy. Conflict may arise when grandparents have a different feeding style and philosophy from the parents and disagreements occur. The most common issue I see is when grandparents start employing a variety of different methods to encourage their grandchildren to eat more. Grandparents love to feed their grandchildren!

My dad is a Vietnam veteran and the second oldest of six siblings who grew up during hard times in the beautiful hills of southern Ohio. He has told me stories of experiencing times when he had barely enough to eat. The winters were long and cold, and he and his siblings were sometimes hungry. His mother worked hard to put enough food on the table to feed all of the children, and it was, at times, rough and uncomfortable.

I love my dad. He is smart, loving, and would sacrifice anything for his grandchildren. However, his childhood experiences have colored his worldview and the way that he feeds others. This is true of some cultures as well. Immigrants to this country may have come from harsh conditions where they experienced hunger in their childhood or even witnessed children starving. For these people, having the luxury of a fat baby or toddler is a gift and blessing. The memory of hunger and the fear that children will not have enough to eat can lead grandparents to overfeed or encourage their grandchildren to ignore their satiety signals.

When my dad picks up the boys from school, he usually arrives prepared with snacks. My boys absolutely love this, and they feel so special. He also cooks delicious meals. Everyone loves Papaw's cooking. I often hear him encouraging the boys to eat a few more bites and offering second or third helpings. He gets so much joy from feeding others.

I will honestly admit that we have butted heads in the past. However, now that my kids are older and we have a good routine and have established intuitive eating habits, I am much more relaxed.

Here are my tips for navigating feeding style differences with family members:

- Be patient.

- Try to understand why your parents or in-laws have the feeding style that they do. Have empathy for their history with food and their bodies.

- If you feel that it is affecting your child negatively, have a gentle conversation with your parents or in-laws about your concerns.

- Try to find a compromise and meet in the middle.

- Take a deep breath! Everything will be okay.

Chapter 17

Common Concerns

The "Picky Eater"

Many parents claim that their child is a "picky eater." Often, they are frustrated because the child won't eat vegetables or eats very little at mealtimes. But what really is a picky eater? Studies have concluded that this behavior in children is part of normal development that decreases over time. They are likely far less picky eaters than parents suspect.

Seemingly "picky" or "fussy" eating may stem from a few different factors. Children that have food neophobia are afraid to try new things. Genetic differences can dictate how sensitive some children are to specific tastes, in particular bitter. People with the "bitter gene" may find bitter foods particularly unpleasant. Many green vegetables are bitter and therefore may be rejected by children with this gene.

What about all these other kids whose parents think are picky? Most of them just aren't hungry (or aren't very hungry) at mealtime. Because they aren't truly hungry, when they sit down and are presented with real foods often consisting of vegetables, they would prefer not to eat. Following are three common causes of decreased appetite at mealtime:

Juice. Drinking juice, milk, or other caloric or sweetened beverages between meals often affects appetite. These beverages contain calories, and calories contribute to satiety, especially for children who are in tune with their bodies. Children should drink only water between meals.

Snacks. Frequent snacking can undermine the consumption of health-promoting foods at mealtime. Feed children if they are hungry, but it doesn't have to be Goldfish crackers and fruit snacks. If you let children play and entertain themselves, you might be surprised that they don't ask for food until the next mealtime and then, miraculously, they happily devour their meal. Experiment with this and see what happens.

Satiety. You have an active toddler with good intuitive eating skills who may not require as many calories as you think to grow and thrive. This is especially apparent during the toddler years when children see the world as one giant playground to discover and explore. They don't stop until it is necessary, and when they do stop to eat, it is just enough to keep going. A toddler's tummy is the size of their fist, and they do not need as much food as a larger person. There are also genetic differences in appetite with some children desiring and requiring fewer calories than others. Trust your child. As long as they are growing and developing normally, trust their eating intuition and their amazing body. You are responsible for providing nutritious food, and they are responsible for choosing how much to put into their gas tank.

Avoid Labeling

When a child is labeled a "picky eater," and this label is repeated over and over in front of the child, it can become part of their identity. This is counterproductive to helping the child develop a broader and more adventurous palate. It can be a self-fulfilling prophecy. What one believes they likely become. Avoid the labeling, see the situation for what it is, and practice the five pillars of healthy eating to guide your child in the principles of intuitive health-promoting eating (page 48).

In summary, in most cases, children who are labeled as "picky eaters" are healthy children who are growing normally. Usually there is not a medical concern or reason to believe that their diet will cause harm. If you follow the principles of intuitive eating, you may find that this is no longer a concern for you. However, even though it is not very common, there may be situations where your child has developed a very restrictive diet and despite all of your efforts, it does not seem to be improving. In addition, if your child is losing weight or not gaining weight appropriately, this may be a sign of a more significant problem. In these cases, they may benefit from professional intervention (see Appendix, page 203).

Overeating, Emotional Eating, and Habitual Eating

As I explained in Part II, some people are more likely to eat when they're not hungry or are more susceptible to emotional eating. These differences are likely rooted in genetics and other learned behaviors. Children who associate food with reward or as a way to relax may develop overeating or emotional eating habits. I want to reemphasize that there is nothing inherently wrong with emotional eating or overeating. There really is no such thing as perfect eating, and everyone will eat outside of hunger and satiety from time to time. However, when it becomes a habit, it might signal a bigger issue. If you feel that your child is starting to use food in this way, the first and most crucial step is to avoid overreacting and/or restricting food. This will likely worsen the situation. The next step is to try to find out if there is a reason why this habit developed. Sometimes it is a simple habit that can be tweaked. Other times it may be a symptom of a deeper emotional need.

When I was in elementary school, I was a latchkey kid and spent several hours at home by myself after school unsupervised. After I finished my homework, I would spend several hours in front of the television eating my snack. I grew up as an only child without any siblings. Honestly, I was bored and didn't have enough to do. I started to associate this afternoon time with eating and taking care of myself. This is very common among children who spend time by themselves in the afternoon. They are likely legitimately hungry after school but combine typical processed snack foods with television watching and a habit emerges.

Processed foods that are high in sugar, salt, and fat can become really fun to eat and some children will quickly learn to enjoy them outside of hunger and satiety. Parents ask me all the time how to deal with this. Limit the amount of processed foods in the house (especially if you have a child that is not yet in school) and create structure around meals and snack time. Continue to offer some of the "snack foods" here and there during the structured meal and snack times, but don't allow it to become a free-for-all. If these foods are particularly alluring to your child, it may be an excellent item to place in their play food drawer (see page 157).

Some children may also have difficulty coping with strong emotions and may inadvertently start using foods to change their moods. I have even encountered young school-age children who ate in response to anxiety and stress. The goal here is not to restrict their diet and shame them for these behaviors, but first of all to recognize and address the emotional component and to help them learn different ways to address these feelings (read more about stress on page 94). And the truth is, we all emotionally eat sometimes. It is normal human behavior.

If you notice that your child seems to be regularly eating more than usual at mealtime, there are several possible explanations or causes. First, they may be experiencing a legitimately increased appetite from a growth spurt. This happened to my older child when he started puberty. The amount of food he was eating was alarming to me, but I knew better than to say anything. When his height shot up and his feet grew by two sizes in a matter of months it all made sense.

Children who become more active with sports or other physical activities will also require more calories. I don't know if there is research evidence to back this up, but I have observed that swimming seems to make children particularly hungry. Children are naturally active, and when they add even more activity to their lives, they will need more calories to support their growth.

Feelings of deprivation or food restriction are another reason why children may overeat. If you think your child may be feeling this way, make changes in your home that align with the five pillars of healthy eating (page 48) and allow your child the space and freedom to tune back into their eating intuition. Remember, the solution is NOT to restrict food; this often makes the problem worse.

Possible reasons for increased food intake:

- Growth spurt

- Pubertal changes

- Increased physical activity from sports/lifestyle change

- Certain medical conditions, such as new-onset diabetes or thyroid disorder

- Certain medications such as steroids

- Temporary metabolic changes from sleep deprivation or stress

- Mood disorders, such as depression or anxiety

- Rebound effect from dieting or being restricted

- Eating disorders, such as bulimia or binge-eating disorder (more on this on page 206)

Signs of overeating in children:

- Seems to be hungry all the time

- Increased preoccupation with food or when the next meal will be

- Constantly asking for snacks

- Sneaking, hiding, or hoarding food

- Eating excessive amounts at mealtime

- Increased snacking between meals

- Eating when bored, stressed, anxious, or sad

Relearning Intuitive Eating

If your child is exhibiting concerning behaviors around food, you may feel that it is too late to change or influence their habits. When a child or any person has restrictions placed around their diet, it can lead to a vicious cycle with food and a disordered relationship with their eating. Often, when parents discover these behaviors, they double down on their efforts to restrict food. I have seen parents place locks on fridges and cabinets, keep food locked in the garage, or punish children for these behaviors. Sadly, this often escalates the problem, these children start and get more and more out of touch with their inner wisdom. It may seem that once this cycle is in place and these behaviors become habitual, it is impossible to relearn intuitive eating, but a two-year pilot study found that even women who have developed eating disorders can learn the skills of intuitive eating.

In my own household, I went through a period when I became overly restrictive about food that I allowed my children to eat. I started to find food wrappers in my son's room and pockets. I also noticed that he was having a difficult time stopping eating certain kinds of foods (particularly the ones I was restricting) when he had access to them.

It took several years, but when I finally understood the connection between dietary restriction and these types of behaviors, it hit me like a ton of bricks. I asked my family to forgive me for those actions that were done with good intent. I asked them to be patient with me as we made the transition into a more flexible, balanced, and intuitive way of eating.

Because I was so used to controlling so much, starting these habits felt incredibly scary to me. I was terrified that my children would only eat processed foods or would overeat routinely if I did not try to control what or how much they ate. It has been an incredible learning experience in trust and appreciation of each child's inner wisdom.

When you are transitioning to a more intuitive way of eating after you have used restrictive feeding patterns in your home, be prepared to employ patience and trust. In the beginning, some behaviors may seem to get worse before they get better. Your child may eat greater quantities of food in general or may just eat more of the foods that were restricted. Take lots of deep breaths and trust that your child will learn to regulate his or her appetite as long as you continue to allow him that space and time to practice. Eventually, these foods will not seem as attractive or exciting as they did when they were being restricted.

Your job is still to provide nutritious and delicious foods along with some play foods within the structure and routine of mealtimes. Once you do this, stay out of the way. Don't judge, criticize, give the "mom" look, or use disapproving body language. This will require practice, and you will not be perfect. It will take some time for your child to trust that you will not swoop in and impose restrictions, but once he does, the past behaviors will fall away. He will trust you after you have shown that you can trust him. This will not happen overnight. I can't tell you how many times I messed up at the beginning of our journey, but I kept the lines of communication open with all my family members. It has taken some time, but I no longer feel the anxiety or worry that I did at the beginning of the journey, and instead, I feel gratitude for learning these skills.

If you are reading this book when you have young children who aren't yet in school, and you feel that you aren't feeding them in a way that supports intuitive eating, you can start making changes without making much fuss. However, if you have an older child and you want to integrate these principles into the way that you feed them, start with a frank conversation about what you have learned and how you would like to change your approach in the house. After I learned more about intuitive eating and knew it was a change that I wanted to make in my house, I called a family meeting with my children and husband, and I discussed what I had learned, what I would change, and why I thought it was necessary. My children were very understanding and excited about the changes (especially the play food drawers). You can have this conversation with your family too. Talk to your child about what foods they would like to have in the house and start including them in menu planning and food preparation. Go through the chapters in Part IV for their age group and begin to implement those habits and behaviors. Keep the communication open as you make these changes and find what works best for your family. Most of all, have fun and give yourself credit for having the courage to make this change that will benefit the entire family!

Conclusion:
The Power of Patience and Persistence

Thank you for taking this journey with me and reading the information in this book. I hope that by now you have learned why giving special attention to your child's eating is essential, how to implement the principles of intuitive eating, and why emphasizing whole plant foods promotes health and longevity in our children. Most of all, I hope that you are feeling more empowered, confident, ready to practice the five pillars of healthy eating (page 48), and practice *your* simple, easy way to raise kids who love to eat healthy.

If at First, You Don't Succeed, Try and Try Again

Just like any skill, learning to feed your family and integrate healthy habits takes practice and some trial and error. Some weeks you are going to feel like Supermom making delicious meals that everyone loves and praises you for. Some days you might not quite hit a home run with everyone and will get some criticism. Other times you may not have time to plan and end up with takeout and fast food. It's okay. We are all just human, and we do the best we can. If you get off track, regroup and start again. Partner up

a parent's guide to intuitive eating

with another mom or mom group in your city or reach out to groups online that have common interests. We simply can't be perfect all the time, and when you get off course, all you have to do is start pointing yourself in the right direction again. Enlist the support of your partner or family member as well as your children. Refresh everybody in the family on the reasons why you choose to eat healthfully and intuitively so that it increases your motivation to start again. You will eventually find your groove, and you will have fewer and fewer moments when you veer off course. Because you don't have the pressure to be 100 percent perfect, you should have no shame or guilt in recognizing when you do veer off course and take measures to course correct.

How You Can Learn More

I hope that you enjoyed this book and gained some great new suggestions and tips for raising your family with a health-promoting way of eating. Before you go, I want to leave you with some helpful resources that you can find in the pages that follow.

It was truly a privilege and honor to write this book for you. I send you off with love, appreciation, and lots of positive energy to guide you on your healthy life. Thanks for being the amazing parent that you are, and never give up on your plantastic journey!

With much love and gratitude,

Dr. Yami

Appendix

In this chapter I will provide information and advice on how to approach a few common medical conditions that can affect appetite and hunger.

Appetite and Illness

Children come into my office most often for short-lived illnesses, such as colds, ear infections, and vomiting and diarrhea. When children are ill, they often lose their appetite. Children who are still nursing will often still nurse for comfort and hydration, and older children will take liquids but may make little effort to eat solid food. Parents become very concerned and worried that the child may lose weight or become weak and not recover rapidly because of this. Ironically, children lose their appetite during illness precisely because the body needs to reserve energy to heal. The body requires quite a bit of energy just to digest food. When we are sick and the body needs to use those energy stores in other ways, our appetite decreases. This is why I counsel parents to not force their children to eat when they are sick. It is supremely important, however, to ensure that your child maintains adequate hydration. Oral rehydration solutions such as Pedialyte have been developed to perfectly match the electrolytes that children need to rehydrate in times of illness, and they are safe for all babies and children. However, for older children, juice or an electrolyte sports drink diluted 50 percent with water will also work. I recommend finding one that does not have artificial dyes in them. Ways to encourage drinking include Popsicles, cold drinks, and offering small sips very frequently.

a parent's guide to intuitive eating

Most illnesses are short and last between five to ten days, and then appetite gradually returns. Some children may lose a little weight when they have these short illnesses, but as soon as they feel better, they bounce back. In fact, don't be surprised if once your child feels better their appetite comes back with a vengeance and they quickly make up for any calories that they missed.

If your child is sick for more than ten days, appears dehydrated, or their appetite does not seem to return, it is best to get them evaluated by their physician.

Chronic Constipation

Constipation is one of my very favorite conditions to treat. It is so gratifying to help a child who has been unable to poop or is having large, painful poops have comfortable, regular bowel movements. This probably has something to do with my personal experience with several decades of chronic constipation and my younger sons struggle with it as well. We both had resolution of our constipation with our dietary change and it was life-changing! The other reason is because it is often pretty simple to fix. I say simple, but not always easy.

Constipation is in the top 10 list of pediatric office visits and may affect up to 30 percent of children. It is defined as having hard, difficult to pass, or very large and infrequent stools. There are children with constipation who have daily bowel movements, but they are small and hard. Some children with chronic constipation develop abdominal pain or nausea when they eat. For some children, chronic constipation can suppress their appetite or cause them to feel full sooner than usual. The diameter of fecal matter can get so large and hard that sometimes children develop rectal fissures with bleeding, rectal tags, or hemorrhoids. Constipation can definitely affect quality of life and become a serious health issue.

The majority of children I treat for constipation fall into three categories (or often a combination of all three):

1. Sensitivity to cow's milk protein. Some of these children are incredibly sensitive and even a bite of dairy can trigger constipation. Getting off all dairy (milk, yogurt, cheese, ice cream, and cream-based foods) might be all they need to start having normal bowel movements.

2. Insufficient fiber intake.

3. Inadequate water intake.

For all children who suffer from constipation, after I collect a thorough history, conduct a physical exam, and rule out other possible physical or serious medical issues, I offer the following tips to parents to help reverse and prevent constipation:

1. Eliminate all dairy (milk, cheese, yogurt, ice cream, and any product that has dairy in the first three ingredients) for at least thirty days to see if it alleviates the constipation. Cheese can be particularly troublesome for some sensitive children. Some parents think that just because their child doesn't like to drink milk that they aren't consuming much dairy, but most kids eat cheese regularly, and dairy is found in many processed foods.

2. Increase fiber intake by focusing on beans, whole grains, and veggies.

3. Add bran and/or ground flaxseed to cereal, oatmeal, smoothies, or muffins.

4. Purée beans into soups and sauces.

5. Ensure adequate water intake throughout the day.

6. Get the child moving regularly and keep them active.

7. Start bowel retraining (see below).

Bowel Retraining

Bowel retraining refers literally to "retraining" the anal sphincter and colon to have normal bowel movements. When children are constipated and have hard stools, they may become desensitized to the feeling of stool in the sigmoid colon, which is the piece of colon in the lower left abdomen that precedes the anus. Another problem is that when stool is very hard or large, it is painful to pass and some younger children start to withhold stool to avoid the pain. This overrides their normal reflex, and the reflex to defecate becomes weaker and weaker until it is almost completely lost. The gastrocolic reflex occurs when the bowels start to contract about fifteen to twenty minutes after a meal. This is a normal pattern for humans and why we often have to visit the toilet after eating a meal. When children are constipated, however, they may not be able to evacuate their bowels, so this intestinal movement causes tummy pain instead. This is one reason why children with constipation have abdominal pain after they eat.

Some children with very long-term constipation may even start leaking stools because they can no longer feel when they have to have a bowel movement. This is called encopresis. Fortunately, it is reversible once the chronic constipation is cured. If kids have been constipated for a long time and are used to withholding because they are afraid of pain, it can take twice as long to retrain the brain and the bowels, so be patient. The most important part of bowel retraining is consistency. Make sure that all caregivers understand the importance of the routine. In addition to continuing the dietary interventions such as avoiding dairy and increasing fiber and water in the diet, implement the following techniques as well. The goal is to ensure that your child is having one to two soft, easy-to-pass bowel movements every day.

Tips for bowel retraining:

- Have your child sit on the toilet fifteen to twenty minutes after breakfast AND dinner in a relaxed manner.

- Use some sort of distraction technique that they only get access to on the potty. Watching a show on the tablet or reading a special book or having a special game are some good ideas.

- Give a nonfood reward for bowel movements. Lots of cheering and clapping, stickers, or access to a special toy.

- Be consistent, and don't give up!

The good news is that if you implement the above and stay persistent and consistent, you are likely to see great improvements in your child's bowel movements until they are no longer suffering from constipation. However, if you have been consistently implementing all of the above for at least one month and your child is still not having daily soft bowel movements or continues to have abdominal pain, please take them to have a formal evaluation by a physician if they have not already. If they are an older child who has had long-term constipation or has encopresis, it may also be beneficial to see a behavioral therapist who specializes in this area.

Attention Deficit and Hyperactivity Disorder (ADHD)

My son was officially diagnosed with ADHD when he was around six years old. I knew before he was born that he was an active child. He would literally turn flips in the womb and moved constantly. As a baby, he was very vocal and did not sleep well. Getting him to nap was a competition sport, and even when he slept well at night he was up by 5 a.m., full of energy and ready to go. He was constantly exploring his environment. He was very curious, and one of his first words was "automatically." In preschool he had difficulty keeping his hands to himself and settling down for circle time and naps. However, his learning was always on track. His teachers would often say, "I am always surprised that he knows the answer because he doesn't seem to be paying attention at all during class." By the time he was in first grade, we decided to try medication to see if it would help his focus in school. We ended up using it for a few years until it seemed that he didn't need it any more. We are lucky that he always had great teachers who worked with him, helped him, and supported him, even during the years when it was more difficult for him to focus. Throughout this time we continued a healthy whole foods plant-based diet and over time I have discovered that he does well with lots of beans, nuts, seeds, and whole plant fats in his diet. We also started a vegan DHA/EPA supplement a few years ago. In addition, I am obsessive about him getting sufficient sleep and exercising adequately. He is now heading into high school, makes honor roll every quarter, is very responsible, is socially motivated, and has always loved school. He still has the advantages of having lots of energy, curiosity, and the love of exploration.

ADHD affects between 8 and 11 percent of children in the United States. ADHD is characterized by distractibility, inattention, impulsivity, and hyperactivity. Raising a child with ADHD can be challenging, tiring, and anxiety-provoking. These children tend to have a lot of energy, and because of their poor impulse control and curiosity, can behave in ways that can be dangerous to them, especially when they are young. Once they are older they might have trouble focusing on topics that are not interesting to them and instead may choose to partake in activities that can be distracting to their classmates. Because of this, they require a lot of attention, both at home and in the classroom.

I believe that their brains and bodies are also very sensitive to substances and medications. It is for this reason that I recommend a diet focused on whole plant foods, foods high in fiber (especially beans), and whole food fats (nuts, seeds, olives, coconut, avocado).

When it comes to eating, children with ADHD may have a couple of different issues to work through. The first is overeating secondary to impulsivity. It is also possible from my anecdotal observations that these children may require greater or more concentrated calories from healthy sources and healthy fats. Their brains really seem to use a lot of energy. Make sure that their meals are balanced with some higher fat plant foods such as nuts or nut butters, and avocado. You may also want to consider an omega-3 DHA/ EPA supplement. It is especially important that you do not restrict these children or make them feel bad for their food choices or the amount of food that they eat. Continue to practice intuitive eating habits in the home, and provide a variety of health-promoting whole foods.

The second issue is that stimulant medications often suppress appetite. This will affect children's hunger drive and, in some cases, can lead to weight loss, poor weight gain, or stunted growth. Because this appetite suppression is caused by external forces and not your child's own intuitive body, ensuring that they are obtaining sufficient calories will require flexibility and adaptability on your part. Provide your child access to a hearty breakfast before they take their morning medication. Most stimulants start to take effect within thirty minutes of ingestion, so if you wait to offer breakfast until after they take their medication, they may not feel hungry enough to eat. Don't panic if they do not eat much or eat very sparingly at lunch. For many children this is when the medication has the strongest effect and their appetite is the lowest. They may have more of an appetite after school or at dinner, but for some children, the appetite may not kick in until a couple of hours before bedtime. This is where I reassure parents that it is okay to be flexible and allow your child to eat a later dinner. It is still very important that you provide health-promoting foods, but include foods that have some density (nuts and nut butters, avocado, coconut, soy) so that they can make up for calories missed at lunch.

General Tips for Children with ADHD

Diet: Emphasize a plant-based diet high in fiber, protein, and healthy fats. Avoid artificial colors, flavors, and additives. This is of PRIME importance. Nutrition is important for all children, but it is especially important with children who have an ADHD diagnosis. Focus on fruits, vegetables, whole grains, beans, and nuts and seeds. All of these foods are rich in fiber and antioxidants, which benefit the brain. Eliminate artificial food dyes, refined sugars, and artificial sugars. Ensure that children who have appetite suppression from stimulants eat breakfast *before* their medication in the morning and be open to allowing them to eat dinner later than usual to allow for hunger to return after the medication has worn off.

Sleep: It is important that kids with ADHD get adequate and restful sleep. Their regular, consistent bedtime routine should include a minimum of nine to ten hours of sleep per night. Keep bedtime and wake times consistent. If your child is on a stimulant, they may have a really hard time falling asleep. If this is the case for your child, talk to your provider. (See Sleep on page 89.)

Physical Activity: These children require a moderate amount of physical activity. I recommend at least sixty minutes of moderate activity per day, but even short bursts of activity throughout the day are great to get the brain fueled and ready to focus. Consider allowing or encouraging participation in individual or team sports.

Supplementation: For my patients with ADHD I recommend a multivitamin that has vitamin D, zinc, and magnesium as well as a vegan omega-3 DHA/EPA supplement and a probiotic. For probiotics, find a product suitable for children that has at least five strains.

Products I like:

Dr. Fuhrman's daily multivitamin—Pixie Vites (chewable and powder for kids), men's or women's (for the teens) (www.DrFuhrman.com)

Complement or Complement Plus (lovecomplement.com)

Dr. Fuhrman Omega 3—DHA/EPA Purity (www.DrFuhrman.com)

Omegazen (find online at amazon.com)

Behavioral Therapy: Most children will benefit from behavioral therapy alone or along with medications and other interventions. Find a therapist you trust who can develop a good rapport with your child.

Open Communication with Your Child's Teachers: Together you can find ways to support your child in the classroom and help him learn. One of my son's teachers let him stand at his desk, and this was very helpful that year. Don't focus on the numbers; you know the truth about your child and how brilliant he or she is.

Emphasize Their Superpowers: Whether it is having lots of energy, creativity, imagination, or artistic skills, highlight all the talents and skills that your child has and allow them to be proud of those qualities.

Frequent Reaffirmation of Love: Children with ADHD can develop low self-esteem because they recurrently feel or hear that they are a problem. This can make them insecure and may even lead them to continue the behaviors because they feel that they will always be that way. Give your child lots of physical affection and words of validation. It really can't be too much.

I have a special place in my heart for children who are diagnosed with ADHD because I know it can be tough for them, their parents, and their teachers. However, these children will grow up to be our future leaders, CEOs, inventors, and innovators. They are able to do amazing things. Our role as parents is to protect their self-esteem and support them through school by optimizing diet and lifestyle habits so that they are able to grow and blossom into the beautiful human beings they are. They are worth every ounce of effort.

When to Seek Professional Help

For some children, intuitive eating, a health-promoting diet, and lifestyle habits won't be sufficient to support healthy growth and development. Children with developmental disorders or other medical conditions that prevent them from eating normally, fall under this category.

Failure to Thrive

Some children do not gain weight normally. This can happen sharply from birth or gradually over time as the growth curve starts to flatten out or take a dip downward. Although there are different ways to define failure to thrive, I define it as a child who is in less than the 2nd percentile for weight and has had a decreased velocity in weight gain that is disproportionate to an increase in length or a child who has had a drop in weight by two major growth percentiles over time regardless of where they started. Failure to thrive affects between 5 and 10 percent of children in the United States.

Three mechanisms can cause failure to thrive:

1. The child is not consuming sufficient calories.

2. The child is not absorbing calories well or losing calories through the GI system or urinary system.

3. The child is burning too many calories (or requires more calories than normal from an increased metabolic rate).

The most common cause of failure to thrive is insufficient intake of calories. The latter two are usually caused by potentially serious medical conditions. If your child is diagnosed with failure to thrive, your pediatrician will investigate the possible reasons with a thorough history and physical. Some children may require lab testing or specialty consults. If your child is also experiencing other issues such as developmental delays or chronic health problems, it is very important to make sure that an underlying condition is not causing the growth issue. This will be best investigated by your child's physician. Children with chronic health problems often benefit from seeing a dietitian to ensure proper growth and weight gain.

If the problem is insufficient calorie intake, a thorough review of the diet is pertinent. Insufficient calorie intake can occur if they do not have access to sufficient food or if they are not eating enough. The most common time that I encounter growth failure is in the first few weeks of life. Sometimes it is because a breastfeeding mother is either not producing sufficient milk, a nursing baby has an ineffective latch or suck that is not prompting the mother to produce sufficient milk, or the baby is unable to transfer it. Once the issue is discovered you can do several things to increase mom's supply or help change the latch.

In older children, failure to thrive may present in toddlerhood. Some children LOVE and prefer non-starchy veggies and fruit and gravitate toward these foods. Although these are incredibly health-promoting and packed with antioxidants, they are also low in calories and high in fiber and can fill up little tummies before the child has consumed enough calories. Some children have very small appetites, eat sparingly, and do not enjoy feeling too full. For children who need to boost calories, the trick would be to add in higher-fat and calorie-dense food, such as nut butters, avocado, coconut, and higher-fat beans, such as soy. I prefer to focus on actual foods rather than liquid meal replacements or between-meal supplements. Once you've made these dietary changes, follow up on their growth frequently until there is sufficient confidence that it will continue on a normal path.

There are also some medical conditions in which children develop an aversion to eating or may develop very restricted diets. Usually these children benefit from visiting a feeding therapist and a dietitian to help with healthy eating behaviors and weight gain.

Pervasive Developmental Disorders

Having a child with autism or another pervasive developmental disorder can be a very stressful full-time job. These children may have aversions to certain foods because of sensory issues. They are also likely to develop very strict preferences. In my experience, many of these children end up with very limited diets of chicken nuggets, cheese pizza, French fries, juice, and hardly anything else. Or they are drinking PediaSure or another liquid supplements throughout the day. This type of diet may come with other adverse effects such as tooth decay, chronic constipation, abdominal pain, skin problems, and extreme behavior problems. For many years, I assumed that this was the best we could do to provide these children with calories. However, now I have come to realize that it really is a vicious cycle. Once we start giving these hyper-palatable foods to these children, they end up craving them more and start to reject other foods. Because parents fear that they won't grow well without them, they keep giving them the very foods that are making them sick, and their kids are exposed to fewer and fewer foods. Although there is currently no cure for autism or other genetic developmental disorders, we do have the ability to optimize lifestyle as much as possible.

Optimizing the way their body feels will also help their mental well-being and emotional balance. It can be a win-win for everyone. However, the road to changing the diet of this type of child can be very challenging and filled with setbacks that a dietitian and a feeding therapist can help with, especially if they have extreme food aversions and restricted diet. My advice for these children is the same as for other children. Focus on fruits, vegetables, whole grains, beans, and nut and seed butters, and start as early as possible. For children who are limited in the textures of foods they eat, find these within plant foods. For older children who are limited to liquids, use plant-based alternatives or homemade formulas. A dietitian can help guide you and find these alternatives. Emphasize leafy greens and beans to get those antioxidants in their bodies.

Your autistic child may also benefit from the supplementation of omega-3 fatty acids, particularly EPA and DHA, which are available in liquid forms. You can also get the ALA form of omega-3 from ground flaxseeds, walnuts, and chia seeds.

I plea that you don't give up. It may take time and a lot of patience, but if you keep at it, you will get your child on a healthier eating path and it will benefit them tremendously.

Eating and Feeding Disorders

Red Flags for Disordered Eating

Despite our best intentions and hard work creating an environment that promotes intuitive eating and healthy body image, there will be some children who start dieting or develop eating disorders. The first thing I want you to know is that it is not your fault. Studies show that there may be genetic susceptibilities that make it more likely for some people to develop an eating disorder. Some eating disorders aren't even really about body size or weight, but a manifestation of obsessive-compulsive disorder. The signs and symptoms may be mixed or subtle. Eating disorders also occur in boys and men, but they may present differently. Girls focus on being thin while boys might focus on decreasing body fat and increasing muscularity. In other words, it's really complicated and beyond the scope of this book to fully explore eating disorders. However, I do want you to be aware of warning signs that your child may be developing an eating disorder so that you can seek professional help as soon as possible.

Signs and symptoms of a possible eating disorder:

- Sudden weight loss or weight gain

- Extreme dissatisfaction with weight, body size, or shape

- Frequent self-checking in mirrors

- Preoccupation with calories or macronutrient content of food

- Language that becomes focused on body size and judging their own or other people's appearance

- Skipping meals and avoiding food

- Eliminating entire food groups (all sugar, all carbs, all fats) or refusing to eat foods they previously liked

- Refusing to eat with the family or making excuses to miss meals

- Excessive exercise or evidence of other forms of purging, such as vomiting, laxatives, or pills

- Evidence of binge-eating indicating consumption of large amounts of food in a short time period

- Mood changes such as depression, anxiety, irritability, withdrawal, and isolation

- Medical problems such as no longer having a period, constipation, diarrhea, abdominal pain, dizziness, fainting, dry skin, and hair loss

I will briefly describe the most common eating disorders so that you are familiar with their symptoms. These disorders have specific medical criteria that help guide practitioners to make a diagnosis and prescribe treatment. One very important thing to keep in mind is that a child does not have to appear emaciated to have an eating disorder. In addition, even if a child does not meet full criteria for the diagnosis of an eating disorder, disordered eating can still cause significant physical and psychological harm.

Anorexia Nervosa

Anorexia is a disorder in which a person will restrict their food intake in order to lose weight or stay at a low weight. People with anorexia may also have purging behaviors, such as vomiting, laxative abuse, and over-exercise (exercising too frequently, too intensely, or for too long). It is three times more common in females than in males. Although anorexia nervosa is rare, it has the highest death rate of any mental illness. The rate of death is six times higher than in the general population. The process of starvation can affect almost every organ system and because of this can have many medical consequences. Anorexia nervosa includes three components:

- Severely restricting food intake so that it leads to extremely low body weight, below what is normal for the individual

- Intense fear of gaining weight or becoming "fat" despite being at an extremely low body weight

- Distortion in the way the individual sees their size or body shape. In other words, people with anorexia may still view themselves as overweight despite being dangerously underweight.

Bulimia Nervosa

Bulimia nervosa is an eating disorder characterized by binge-eating followed by severe and inappropriate compensatory behaviors such as fasting, laxative or diuretic abuse, vomiting, or over-exercise. Similar to those with anorexia, those with bulimia are greatly affected by their body weight and shape. There is no weight criteria for diagnosing bulimia. It is possible to have severe bulimia and not be overly thin. Bulimia is associated with a higher frequency of self-harm, including suicide attempts. As with anorexia, this disorder comes with many medical complications, and the death rate is higher than in the general population.

Binge-Eating Disorder

Binge-eating disorder is often associated with other mental health conditions, such as depression, and it tends to include large weight fluctuations. People with this disorder tend to eat large amounts of food in short periods of time in which they feel lack of control and eat until they are uncomfortably full, often when they are not physically hungry. They often feel guilty and ashamed after these episodes. Associated compensatory behaviors don't usually follow these binge episodes, but people with binge-eating disorder usually feel dissatisfied with their weight and appearance.

I want to touch upon a couple of lesser-known eating/feeding disorders that can cause failure to thrive in children or teens. These disorders definitely necessitate medical attention and support from professionals, who can help ensure that these children grow properly.

Avoidant Restrictive Food Intake Disorder (ARFID)

Children with this disorder have a very restrictive diet elicited by fear or disgust of food. They may lose weight or have trouble gaining weight because they do not enjoy eating. They may also be very sensitive to the sensations of food and have aversions to a wide variety of textures and flavors. These children are not focused on size or weight. Because this is a rare disorder, it will require evaluation by a medical professional and a team of professionals to ensure proper treatment.

Orthorexia Nervosa

People with orthorexia are not usually preoccupied with their weight or body size but develop an obsession with eating a diet that they consider healthy. People with orthorexia may eliminate several food groups or types of food that do not fit their criteria of healthfulness or purity. It becomes a disorder when it starts interfering with normal social functioning and causes anxiety. Although orthorexia may not affect weight, it will cause a disordered relationship with food. If you feel that your child has developed symptoms of orthorexia, a therapist or specialist in eating disorders can help.

If your child is exhibiting symptoms of any of these eating disorders, please see a medical professional for an evaluation. The sooner you seek and receive help for your child, the better.

Resources

Books

Intuitive Eating and Health at Every Size

Body Respect: What Conventional Health Books Get Wrong, Leave Out, and Just Plain Fail to Understand About Weight by Linda Bacon and Lucy Aphramor

Health at Every Size: The Surprising Truth about Your Weight by Linda Bacon

Intuitive Eating: A Revolutionary Program That Works by Evelyn Tribole and Elyse Resch

The Intuitive Eating Workbook: Ten Principles for Nourishing a Healthy Relationship with Food by Evelyn Tribole and Elyse Resch

The Intuitive Eating Workbook for Teens: A Non-Diet, Body Positive Approach to Building a Healthy Relationship with Food by Elyse Resch

Body Image and Body Acceptance

The Body Is Not an Apology : The Power of Radical Self-Love by Sonya Renee Taylor

Celebrate Your Body (and Its Changes, Too!): The Ultimate Puberty Book for Girls by Sonya Renee Taylor and Bianca I. Laureano

No Weigh! A Teen's Guide to Positive Body Image, Food, and Emotional Wisdom by Signe Darpinian, Wendy Sterling, and Shelley Aggarwal

Eating Disorders

Help Your Teenager Beat an Eating Disorder by James Lock and Daniel Le Grange

Feeding Children

Child of Mine: Feeding with Love and Good Sense by Ellyn Satter

Helping Your Child with Extreme Picky Eating: A Step-by-Step Guide for Overcoming Selective Eating, Food Aversion, and Feeding Disorders by Katja Rowell, MD and Jenny McGlothlin, MS

Your Child's Weight: Helping without Harming by Ellyn Satter

Plant-Based Nutrition

The China Study: Startling Implications for Diet, Weight Loss, and Long-Term Health by T. Colin Campbell and Thomas M. Campbell II

Disease-Proof Your Child: Feeding Kids Right by Joel Fuhrman

Eat to Live: The Amazing Nutrient-Rich Program for Fast and Sustained Weight Loss by Joel Fuhrman

Forks Over Knives Family: Every Parent's Guide to Raising Healthy, Happy Kids on a Whole-Food, Plant-Based Diet by Alona Pulde, MD and Matthew Lederman, MD

The Happy Herbivore Guide to Plant-Based Living by Lindsay S. Nixon

The Healthiest Diet on the Planet by John McDougall, MD

Vegan for Her: The Woman's Guide to Being Healthy and Fit on a Plant-Based Diet by Virginia Messina and JL Fields

The Vegan Starter Kit: Everything You Need to Know about Plant-Based Eating by Neal D. Barnard, MD

Your Complete Vegan Pregnancy: Your All-in-One Guide to a Healthy, Holistic, Plant-Based Pregnancy by Reed Mangels

Chronic Disease Prevention and Reversal

The Alzheimer's Solution: A Breakthrough Program to Prevent and Reverse the Symptoms of Cognitive Decline at Every Age by Dean Sherzai and Ayesha Sherzai

Dr. Neal Barnard's Program for Reversing Diabetes: The Scientifically Proven System for Reversing Diabetes Without Drugs by Neal D. Barnard and Bryanna Clark Grogan

How Not to Die: Discover the Foods Scientifically Proven to Prevent and Reverse Disease by Michael Greger and Gene Stone

The Longevity Diet: Discover the New Science Behind Stem Cell Activation and Regeneration to Slow Aging, Fight Disease, and Optimize Weight by Valter Longo

The Plant-Based Solution: America's Healthy Heart Doc's Plan to Power Your Health by Joel Kahn

Prevent and Reverse Heart Disease: The Revolutionary, Scientifically Proven, Nutrition-Based Cure by Caldwell B. Esselstyn

Undo It!: How Simple Lifestyle Changes Can Reverse Most Chronic Diseases by Dean Ornish, MD and Anne Ornish

The Vegan Heart Doctor's Guide to Reversing Heart Disease, Losing Weight, and Reclaiming Your Life by Heather Shenkman, MD

Cookbooks

The College Vegan Cookbook: 145 Affordable, Healthy & Delicious Plant-Based Recipes by Heather Nicholds

Forks Over Knives -The Cookbook: Over 300 Recipes for Plant-Based Eating All Through the Year by Del Sroufe and Isa Chandra Moskowitz

The Happy Herbivore Cookbook: Over 175 Delicious Fat-Free and Low-Fat Vegan Recipes by Lindsay S. Nixon

Plant-Powered Families: Over 100 Kid-Tested, Whole-Foods Vegan Recipes by Dreena Burton

The Prevent and Reverse Heart Disease Cookbook : Over 125 Delicious, Life-Changing, Plant-Based Recipes by Anne Crile Esselstyn and Jane Esselstyn

Unprocessed: How to Achieve Vibrant Health and Your Ideal Weight by Chef AJ and Glen Merzer

The Vegan 8: 100 Simple, Delicious Recipes Made with 8 Ingredients or Less by Brandi Doming

Vive Le Vegan! Simple, Delectable Recipes for the Everyday Vegan Family by Dreena Burton

Other Books of Interest

The Blue Zones: 9 Lessons for Living Longer from the People Who've Lived the Longest (second edition) by Dan Buettner

First Bite: How We Learn to Eat by Bee Wilson

Mindless Eating: Why We Eat More Than We Think by Brian Wansink

The Secret Life of Fat: The Science Behind the Body's Least Understood Organ and What It Means for You by Sylvia Tara

Parenting

The Happiest Baby on the Block : The New Way to Calm Crying and Help Your Newborn Baby Sleep Longer by Harvey Karp

Websites

Doctor Yami: www.doctoryami.com

Eating Disorders Tool Kit: www.nationaleatingdisorders.org/parent-toolkit

Evidence-Based Nutrition videos: www.nutritionfacts.org

Health at Every Size: www.haescommunity.com

Association for Size Diversity and Health: www.sizediversityandhealth.org

Intuitive Eating: www.intuitiveeating.org

Kelly Mom, Parenting and Breastfeeding: www.kellymom.com

La Leche League International (Breastfeeding Support): www.llli.org

Signing Time: www.signingtime.com

UK-based feeding guide for plant-based children "Eating Well: Vegan Infants and Under 5's": www.firststepsnutrition.org/eating-well-early-years

Veggie Fit Kids: www.veggiefitkids.com

Cooking Blogs

Dreena Burton: www.plantpoweredkitchen.com

Fork and Beans: www.forkandbeans.com

The Full Helping: www.thefullhelping.com

Minimalist Baker: www.minimalistbaker.com

Oh She Glows: www.ohsheglows.com

Vegan Richa: www.veganricha.com

Selected Bibliography

Carbonneau, Eise, Catherine Begin, Simone Lemieux, et al. "A Health at Every Size Intervention Improves Intuitive Eating and Diet Quality in Canadian Women." *Clinical Nutrition* 36, no. 3 (June 2017): 747–54.

Ciampolini, Mario, H. David Lovell-Smith, Timothy Kenealy, et al. "Hunger Can Be Taught: Hunger Recognition Regulates Eating and Improves Energy Balance." *International Journal of General Medicine* 6 (June 2013): 465–78.

Dhana, Klodian, Jess Haines, Gang Liu, et al. "Association between Maternal Adherence to Healthy Lifestyle Practices and Risk of Obesity in Offspring: Results from Two Prospective Cohort Studies of Mother-Child Pairs in the United States." *BMJ* 362, no. k2486 (July 2018). http://dx.doi.org/10.1136/bmj.k2486.

Faith, Myles S., Kelley S. Scanlon, Leann L. Birch, et al. "Parent-Child Feeding Strategies and Their Relationships to Child Eating and Weight Status." *Obesity Research* 12, no 11 (November 2004): 1711–22.

Hawks, Steven, Hala Madanat, Jaylyn Hawks, et al. "The Relationship Between Intuitive Eating and Health Indicators Among College Women." *American Journal of Health Education* 36, no. 6 (2005): 331–36.

Herle, Moritz, Alison Fildes, Fruhling Rijsdijk, et al. "The Home Environment Shapes Emotional Eating." *Child Development* 89, no. 4 (July 2018): 1423–34.

Hirotsu, Camila, Sergio Tufik, and Monica Levy Andersen. "Interactions between Sleep, Stress, and Metabolism: From Physiological to Pathological Conditions." *Sleep Science* 8, no. 3 (November 2015): 143–52.

Hughes, Sheryl O. and Alexis C. Frazier-Wood. "Satiety and the Self-Regulation of Food Take in Children: A Potential Role for Gene-Environmental Interplay." *Current Obesity Reports* 5, no. 1 (March 2016): 81–7.

Humphrey, Lauren, Dawn Clifford, and Michelle Neyman Morris. "Health at Every Size College Course Reduces Dieting Behaviors and Improves Intuitive Eating, Body Esteem, and Anti-Fat Attitudes." *Journal of Nutrition Education and Behavior* 47, no. 4 (2015): 354–60.

Knutson, Kristen L., Karine Spiegel, Plamen Penev, et al. "The Metabolic Consequences of Sleep Deprivation." *Sleep Medicine Reviews* 11, no. 3 (June 2007): 163–78.

Kral, Tanja V. E., David B. Allison, Leann L. Birch, et al. "Caloric Compensation and Eating in the Absence of Hunger in 5- to 12-Y-Old Weight-Discordant Siblings." *American Journal of Clinical Nutrition* 96, no. 3 (September 2012): 574–83.

Lam, Jason. "Picky Eating in Children." *Frontiers in Pediatrics* 3, no. 41 (May 2015). http://doi.org/10.3389/fped.2015.00041.

Loth, Katie A., Richard F. MacLehose, Jayne A. Fulkerson, et al. "Are Food Restriction and Pressure-to-Eat Parenting Practices Associated with Adolescent Disordered Eating Behaviors?" *International Journal of Eating Disorders* 47, no. 3 (April 2014): 310–14.

Lowes, Jacinta and Marika Tiggemann. "Body Dissatisfaction, Dieting Awareness and the Impact of Parental Influence in Young Children." *British Journal of Health Psychology* 8 (May 2003): 135–47.

McNally, Janet, Siobhan Hugh-Jones, Samantha Caton, et al. "Communicating Hunger and Satiation in the First 2 Years of Life: A

a parent's guide to intuitive eating

Systematic Review." *Maternal and Child Nutrition* 12, no. 2 (April 2016): 205–28.

Monsivais, Pablo, Anju Aggarwal, and Adam Drewnowski. "Time Spent on Home Preparation and Indicators of Healthy Eating." *American Journal of Preventive Medicine* 47, no. 6 (December 2014): 796–802.

Patrick, Heather, Theresa A. Nicklas, Sheryl O. Hughes, et al. "The Benefits of Authoritative Feeding Style: Caregiver Feeding Styles and Children's Food Consumption Patterns." *Appetite* 44 (2005): 243–49.

Pervanidou, Panagiota and George P. Chrousos. "Metabolic Consequences of Stress During Childhood and Adolescence." *Metabolism* 61, no. 5 (May 2012): 611–19.

Popkin, Barry M. and Kiyah J. Duffey. "Does Hunger and Satiety Drive Eating Anymore? Increasing Eating Occasions and Decreasing Time between Eating Occasions in the United States." *American Journal of Clinical Nutrition* 91, no. 5 (May 2010): 1342–47.

Powell, Faye C., Claire V. Farrow, and Caroline Meyer. "Food Avoidance in Children. The Influence of Maternal Feeding Practices and Behaviours." *Appetite* 57, no. 3 (December 2011): 683–92.

Richards, P. Scott, Sabree Crowton, Michael E. Berrett, et al. "Can Patients with Eating Disorders Learn to Eat Intuitively? A 2-year Pilot Study." *Eating Disorders* 25, no. 2 (March 2017): 99–113.

Rodgers, Rachel F., Susan J. Paxton, Robin Massey, et al. "Maternal Feeding Practices Predict Weight Gain and Obesogenic Eating Behaviors in Young Children: A Prospective Study." *International Journal of Behavioral Nutrition and Physical Activity* 10, no. 24 (2013): 1–10. http://www.ijbnpa.org/content/10/1/24.

Sabate, Joan and Michelle Wien. "Vegetarian Diets and Childhood Obesity Prevention." *American Journal and Clinical Nutrition* 91, no. 5 (May 2010): 1525S–1529S.

Schaefer, Julie T., and Amy Magnuson. "A Review of Interventions that Promote Eating by Internal Cues." *Journal of the Academy of Nutrition and Dietetics* 114, no. 5 (May 2014): 734–60.

Smith, TeriSue, and Steven R. Hawks. "Intuitive Eating, Diet Composition, and the Meaning of Food in Healthy Weight Promotion." *American Journal of Health Education* 37, no. 3 (January 2013): 130–36.

Steinsbekk, Silje, Edward D. Barker, Clare Llewellyn, et al. "Emotional Feeding and Emotional Eating: Reciprocal Processes and the Influence of Negative Affectivity." *Child Development* 89, no. 4 (July 2018): 1234–46.

Stifter, Cynthia, Stephanie Anzman-Frasca, Leann L. Birch, et al. "Parent Use of Food to Soothe Infant/Toddler Distress and Child Weight Status. An Exploratory Study." *Appetite* 57, no. 3 (December 2011): 693–99.

Tylka, Tracy L., Julie C. Lumeng, and Ihuoma U. Eneli. "Maternal Intuitive Eating as a Moderator of the Association between Concern about Child Weight and Restrictive Child Feeding." *Appetite* 95 (December 2015): 158–65.

Conversions

Volume

U.S.	U.S. Equivalent	Metric
1 tablespoon (3 teaspoons)	½ fluid ounce	15 milliliters
¼ cup	2 fluid ounces	60 milliliters
⅓ cup	3 fluid ounces	80 milliliters
½ cup	4 fluid ounces	120 milliliters
⅔ cup	5 fluid ounces	160 milliliters
¾ cup	6 fluid ounces	180 milliliters
1 cup	8 fluid ounces	240 milliliters
2 cups	16 fluid ounces	480 milliliters

Weight

U.S.	Metric
½ ounce	15 grams
1 ounce	30 grams
2 ounces	60 grams
¼ pound	115 grams
⅓ pound	150 grams
½ pound	225 grams
¾ pound	340 grams
1 pound	450 grams

Temperature

Fahrenheit (°F)	Celsius (°C)
70°F	20°C
100°F	40°C
120°F	50°C
130°F	55°C
140°F	60°C
150°F	65°C
160°F	70°C
170°F	75°C
180°F	80°C
190°F	90°C
200°F	95°C
220°F	105°C
240°F	115°C
260°F	125°C
280°F	140°C
300°F	150°C
325°F	165°C
350°F	175°C
375°F	190°C
400°F	200°C
425°F	220°C
450°F	230°C
500°F	260°C

a parent's guide to intuitive eating

Index

Acknowledgments

First of all, I would like to thank Ulysses Press and Casie Vogel for believing in me and inviting me to write this book. It is a dream come true, and I am so grateful to have this opportunity. I would also like to thank the various editors that have helped me polish this work. Renee Rutledge, I am so grateful for your patience and attention to detail! Editing is definitely an art form and I appreciate your expertise so much!

Many thanks to my gracious mother-in-love, Janey Lancaster, who was always available to read sections of this book, give me great feedback, and help me with my grammar. I'm lucky to be related to an English teacher.

Many thanks to my parents, Griselda and Rodney, for being the most amazing grandparents ever. Thanks for taking such great care of my kids and feeding them with love.

Endless thanks to my amazing husband, Brad, who was very patient and supportive with me throughout the writing of this book. I missed many family weekend trips so that I could have enough time and space to think and write. I found that for me, the writing process requires lots of free time to think and organize my thoughts, and I am forever grateful that he allowed me this luxury.

I am very thankful to my children for giving me the amazing experience of motherhood and for all the love they shower me with despite all my mistakes and flaws.

a parent's guide to intuitive eating

So much gratitude to my right-hand woman, Alejandra Parra. Thank you for running the office, solving problems before I even knew they existed, and your support. You are the best!!

I couldn't have come this far without my amazing mastermind partner, and real-life Rockstar, Angela Soffe, and her support, inspiration, and encouragement. Thank you for making me laugh during my times of doubt and struggle and for believing in me when I didn't believe in myself.

I also am forever indebted to all of the coaches and teachers I have had throughout my journey.

Many thanks to librarians Mary Beth McAteer from Virginia Mason Medical Center and Mary Giovanni from Pacific Northwest University of Health Sciences for help in gathering articles for me.

I would be amiss if I did not thank the many pioneers that came before me and helped pave the way for Intuitive Eating, Health at Every Size, body positivity, and plant-based nutrition. Your courage, passion, and dedication have created a solid foundation that has positively impacted so many lives. Thank you for all that you do!

Finally, I thank all of my patients and their parents for trusting me with their care and allowing me the opportunity to have my dream job. I am honored and forever grateful to be your pediatrician. I love you all so much!

About the Author

Dr. Yami is a board-certified pediatrician, national board-certified health and wellness coach, author, and professional speaker. She is a passionate promoter of healthy lifestyles, especially the power of plant-based diets for the prevention of chronic disease. She founded VeggieFitKids.com, where she provides information on plant-based diets for children and hosts the podcast *Veggie Doctor Radio*.

She obtained a certificate in plant-based nutrition in 2013, is a certified Food for Life Instructor, and is a Jack Canfield Success Principles Certified Trainer. She is a fellow of the American Academy of Pediatrics and a member of the American College of Lifestyle Medicine.

Dr. Yami owns Nourish Wellness, a pediatric micro-practice in Yakima, WA, where she lives with her husband and two active sons. You can find out more about Dr. Yami at DoctorYami.com.